Many thanks for all your help in precepting our FNP students!

The NP Faculty at UVM

October 1998

OBSTETRIC AND GYNECOLOGIC DERMATOLOGY

MARTIN M BLACK

MD FRCP FRCPATH

Consultant Dermatologist and Senior Lecturer Chairman
Department of Dermatopathology
St. John's Institute of Dermatology
St Thomas' Hospital
London, UK

MARILYNNE McKAY

MD

Professor of Dermatology and Gynecology/Obstetrics
Emory University of Medicine
Atlanta, USA

PETER R BRAUDE

MBBCh MA PhD FRCOG

Professor of Obstetrics and Gynecology Chairman and
Head of Department United Medical and Dental Schools of
Guy's and St Thomas' Hospitals
London, UK

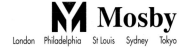

London   Philadelphia   St Louis   Sydney   Tokyo

Dedications

To my wife, Aniko.

M M Black

To a special mentor, the late Eduard G. Friedrich, Jr; my husband, Ronald S. Hosek; and my patients, who have taught me so much.

M McKay

To Beatrice, Philip and Richard, and to a certain house in Ireland which made this all possible.

P R Braude

Copyright © 1995 Times Mirror International Publishers Ltd.

Published in 1995 by Mosby–Wolfe, an imprint of Times Mirror International Publishers Limited.

Printed in Italy by G. Canale & C. S.p.A. - Borgaro T.se - TURIN

Reprinted in 1996 and 1997.

Reprinted in 1998 by Mosby International

ISBN 0 7234 2009 2

For full details of all Mosby International titles please write to Mosby International, Lynton House, 7–12 Tavistock Square, London WC1H 9LB, UK.

Project Manager:	Alison Taylor
Development Editor:	Jennifer Prast
Designer:	Judith Gauge
Layout Artist:	Jonathan Brenchley
Cover Design:	Lara Last
Illustration:	Marion Tasker
Production:	Cathy Martin
Index:	Dr M McKay Anita Reid
Publisher:	Richard Furn

Contents

PREFACE

This text is the first ever to focus specifically on the full range of dermatologic problems encountered in obstetric and gynecologic practice. For the first time, sections on the vulva, inflammatory vulvar disease and vulvar tumors have been combined with chapters related to the obstetric manifestations of skin disease. This profusely illustrated color atlas presents numerous examples of common and unusual disorders. The opportunity to compare images of similar-appearing skin problems in the clinic or at the bedside will be appreciated by consulting dermatologists and non-dermatologists alike.

The authors have distilled their considerable experience to present a basic, sensible approach to a complex subject. Overview chapters explain major diagnostic issues clearly, using current terminology. The well referenced text covers differential diagnosis, complications, and the management of dermatoses in pregnancy and vulvar disorders, as well as common skin conditions that may be affected by pregnancy. The text outlines in detail practical suggestions for therapy, including patient information sheets for the major vulvar dermatoses to copy and give to the patient. An appendix on differential diagnosis of vulvar ulcers helps the clinician choose an appropriate and cost-effective workup before starting therapy.

We are proud of the combined effort — we think that this book will be a useful reference for all clinicians who care about womens' health.

Martin M Black
Marilynne McKay
Peter R Braude

CONTRIBUTORS

Neil N M Buchanan MBChB FRCP
Honorary Consultant Physician,
St Thomas' Hospital, London, UK

Diana Hamilton Fairley MBBS MRCOG MD
Lecturer in Obstetrics and Gynaecology,
UMDS, Guy's and St Thomas' Hospital,
London, UK

M John Hare MA, MD, FRCOG
Consultant Obstetrician and Gynaecologist,
Hinchingbrooke Healthcare Trust,
Huntington, Cambridgeshire, UK

Christine Harrington MD FRCP
Consultant Dermatologist,
Royal Hallamshire Hospital,
Sheffield, UK

Ira R Horowitz MD FACOG FACS
Associate Professor,
Director of Gynecologic Oncology,
Emory University School of Medicine,
Atlanta, Georgia, USA

Graham R V Hughes MD FRCP
Consultant Rheumatologist,
The Rayne Institute,
St. Thomas' Hospital, London, UK

Rachel E Jenkins BSc MRCP
Senior Registrar,
St John's Institute of Dermatology,
St Thomas' Hospital, London, UK

Michael Katesmark MA FRCS MRCOG
Senior Registrar, Department of Obstetrics
and Gynaecology,
The Lewisham Hospital NHS Trust,
Lewisham, London, UK

Sian Kerslake MB, BCH, FRCS(Ed), MRCOG
Senior Registrar,
Farnborough Hospital,
Farnborough, Kent, UK

Munther A Khamashta MD PhD
Deputy Director of the Lupus Arthritis
Research Unit,
The Rayne Institute,
St Thomas' Hospital, London, UK

Pauline Marren MRCP
Senior Registrar in Dermatology
Oxford Radcliffe Hospitals, Oxford, UK

John M Monaghan MB FRCS FRCOG
Director of Gynaecological Oncology
Services,
Senior Lecturer in Gynaecological Oncology,
University of Newcastle upon Tyne, UK

Sallie M Neill MB ChB MRCP
Consultant Dermatologist,
St John's Dermatology Centre,
St Thomas' Hospital, London, UK and
Consultant Dermatologist,
St Peter's Hospital,
Chertsey, Surrey, UK

C Marjorie Ridley MA FRCP
Honorary Consultant Dermatologist,
St Thomas' Hospital, London, UK

Barbara Rock MD
Assistant Professor of Dermatology,
Emory University School of Medicine,
Atlanta, Georgia, USA

Jeff K Shornick MD
Associate Professor of Dermatology,
University of Washington School of
Medicine,
Staff Physician, Group Health
Cooperative of Puget Sound,
Seattle, Washington, USA

Catherine J M Stephens MBBS MRCP
Consultant Dermatologist,
Poole Hospital NHS Trust,
Poole, Dorset, UK

Alison Taylor MBBS, MRCOG
Lecturer in Obstetrics and Gynaecology,
UMDS Guy's and St Thomas' Hospital,
London, UK

Fenella Wojnarowska FRCP
Consultant Dermatologist and Senior
Clinical Lecturer,
Department of Dermatology,
Oxford Radcliffe Hospitals, Oxford, UK

1.
Hormonal Changes in Pregnancy, the Menarche, and Menopause

Diana Hamilton-Fairley & Peter Braude

INTRODUCTION

This chapter summarizes the hormonal changes that occur during puberty, the menstrual cycle, pregnancy, and the menopause, and how these changes affect the skin physiologically.

All children go through the bewildering hormonal changes that the transition from child to adult necessitates. However, it is only the female who will continue to experience a changing hormonal milieu – either cyclically, with the monthly production of an egg followed by menses, or the effects of pregnancy if conception takes place. Then, for the last third of their lives, women face the consequences of a reduction in estrogen levels following the menopause. Although the hormonal events immediately preceding the menopause are turbulent, once the climacteric is reached, it too may cause its problems.

Most women are aware of the changes taking place in their skin at these different stages in their lives.

HYPOTHALAMIC–PITUITARY AXIS

Before discussing each phase of hormonal change in detail, it is important to understand the inter-relationship between the hypothalamus, the pituitary gland, and the ovary.

Situated above the pituitary gland, the hypothalamus initiates the release of the polypeptides that regulate ovarian function. The ovary cannot produce mature fertile oocytes (eggs) if the signals from the pituitary gland never start or cease, or are disordered. The female reproductive cycle is precisely regulated via biologic feedback mechanisms from the ovary, which alter the activity of the hypothalamus and pituitary. Normal physiologic changes in the functioning of the hypothalamic–pituitary axis result in the hormonal changes that occur during the four main reproductive endocrine phases of a woman's life – puberty, menstruation, pregnancy, and the menopause.

PUBERTY

Puberty describes the physiologic, morphologic, and behavioral changes that occur in a child as the gonads mature from the infantile to the adult state. Puberty affects most of the organs of the body in both sexes, but this chapter discusses only the changes occurring in girls.

Physiologic changes can be divided into two main groups – growth and hormonal. Although these changes start at different chronologic ages in different individuals, there is a similar sequence of events. The start of puberty seems to be strongly weight-related, with the mean body weight being 47kg at menarche. Although the age of menarche has decreased from 17 years in 1840 to 13.5 years in the 1940s, and is now 12.5 years in the USA, the mean body weight at menarche seems to have remained constant.

GROWTH SPURT

The adolescent growth spurt is an acceleration of growth in most skeletal dimensions. The peak height velocity (PHV) is 9–10cm per year and lasts for about two years. There is no difference in the PHV of girls and boys, and both sexes grow between 25 and 28cm during puberty. However, girls start their growth spurt two years earlier than boys, at which time they are 10cm shorter than when boys start theirs. This accounts for the difference in adult height between the sexes.

This large increase in height is mediated by an increase in growth hormone (GH) production by the pituitary gland. The greatest increase in the frequency and amplitude of GH takes place at night in a similar fashion to luteinizing hormone (LH) pulses (**1.1**).

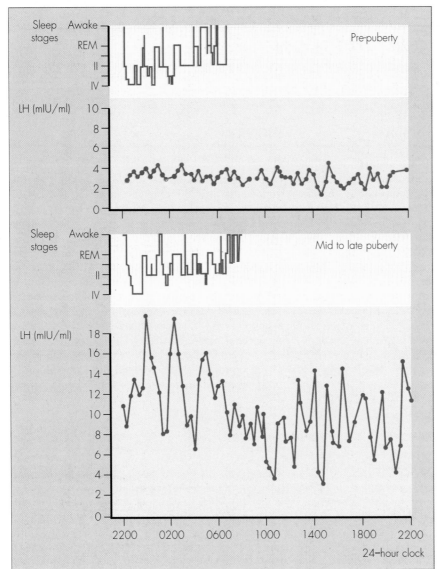

1.1 Luteinizing hormone levels during puberty. Changes in the pulse frequency and amplitude of luteinizing hormone during puberty.

HORMONAL CHANGES

The hormonal changes of puberty have two main effects – the maturation of the ovary so that reproduction can take place, and the development of secondary sexual characteristics (breasts; axillary and pubic hair).

During childhood, serum levels of the gonadotrophins – LH and follicle-stimulating hormone (FSH) – are low. During early to mid-puberty, however, there is a striking increase in the magnitude and frequency of LH pulses at night during sleep (**1.1**). In late puberty, there is an increase in magnitude during the day, but not as much as at night. It is only when puberty is complete that the LH pulses lose their diurnal variation and settle into an adult pattern. This consists of a pulse approximately every 90 minutes during the follicular phase, and between 120 and 180 minutes in the luteal phase.

These events are probably initiated by the maturation of the hypothalamus and the onset of secretion of gonadotrophin-releasing hormone (GnRH). It is,

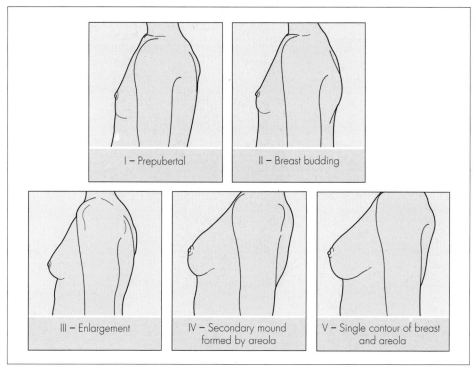

1.2 Breast development. The Tanner stages I–V of breast development.

I – Prepubertal

II – Breast budding

III – Enlargement

IV – Secondary mound formed by areola

V – Single contour of breast and areola

however, impossible to prove the exact sequence of events initiating puberty since the experiments required would be unethical in humans.

The increase in both LH and FSH has a trophic effect on the ovary, and stimulates the production of estradiol. The primordial follicles, present from birth, begin to mature into antral follicles lined by granulosa cells. The process of maturation takes about 10 weeks[1]. Luteinizing hormone acts mainly on the theca cells which surround the follicles, causing them to produce testosterone. This is then converted to estradiol in the granulosa cells by an aromatase under the influence of FSH.

The increase in estradiol secretion leads to breast development. This is divided into five stages, taking about four years to complete (**1.2**). Menstruation usually occurs once breast development is quite well advanced – between stages III and IV.

Several other changes also occur, which are particularly important in understanding physiologic changes in the skin. The first is adrenarche. This is an increase in the production of adrenal androgens, dehydroepiandrosterone (DHEA) and its sulfate (DHEAS), which starts at about eight years of age and

continues until 13–15 years of age in both sexes. This increase is thought to stimulate the development of axillary and pubic hair, as hair growth and changes in sebum secretion are predominantly modulated by androgens in both sexes. Pubic and axillary hair usually starts developing before the breasts, because of the increase in adrenal androgens, but reaches the mature stage at around the same time. The testosterone level increases in girls, as in boys, under the influence of LH, but most of the testosterone is converted into estradiol.

During puberty, the concentration of the main binding protein of the sex hormones (sex hormone-binding globulin, SHBG) declines in both sexes, despite the increase in estradiol concentrations in girls[2,3]. Sex hormone-binding globulin has a greater affinity for testosterone than for estradiol, with the result that, in most girls, more than 90% of circulating testosterone is bound to SHBG, thus limiting the effect that testosterone may have peripherally. The decrease in SHBG seems to be mediated by an increase in insulin concentration, which has been demonstrated in both sexes[4].

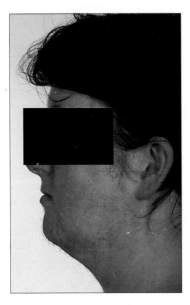

1.3 Polycystic ovary syndrome. Facial hirsutism associated with polycystic ovary syndrome.

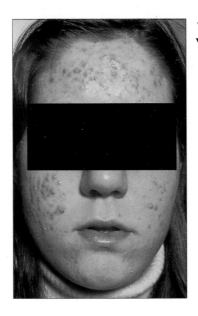

1.4 Acne vulgaris.

POLYCYSTIC OVARY SYNDROME

There is a group of girls who produce an excess of testosterone accompanied by morphologic changes in their ovaries – a phenomenon known as polycystic ovaries (PCO). They are often those girls who never establish regular menstruation and who have increased hair growth, usually of a male pattern, with an abdominal escutcheon, moustache, or other facial hair growth (**1.3**). They may also develop acne. Indeed, it has been shown that most girls with acne and/or hirsutism have polycystic ovary syndrome[5]. These girls also have higher insulin concentrations and lower SHBG concentrations than their weight-matched contemporaries[6].

A lower SHBG concentration, together with an increased circulating testosterone concentration, will lead to an increased free testosterone concentration. It is the fraction of free testosterone which is thought to be active peripherally on the skin, sebaceous glands, and hair follicles.

ACNE

Testosterone has major effects on the hair follicle and sebum secretion. Acne vulgaris (**1.4**) and hirsutism are never seen in prepubertal children with normal adrenal function, providing further evidence that puberty-related changes trigger these events.

Acne is the result of one or more of the following processes in the pilosebaceous follicle:
• Inflammation;
• Overactivity;
• Disturbed cornification;
• Increased microbial colonization[7].
The pilosebaceous gland becomes more differentiated, increases in size, and changes its sebum composition. These changes are most marked on the scalp and around the nose, chin, and cheeks, as well as on the upper chest and back. Acne tends to reach a peak during puberty and before sexual maturity. It is therefore thought that the adrenal glands provide the initial stimulus[8,9].

The principal hormone involved in women is testosterone. Free testosterone enters the basal sebocytes and is converted within the cytoplasm by 5-α-reductase to 5-α-dihydrotestosterone (DHT). This new compound binds to a specific cytosolic receptor protein and, in the form of an androgen-receptor complex, it is then transported into the nucleus of the cell. Here, signals are produced that allow the biosynthesis of other factors that control sebocyte function. These factors also control mechanisms that include the production of 3-α-androstenediol glucuronide from DHT.

The proliferation of the sebaceous glands and their differentiation are mainly dependent on the amount of androgens taken up by the cell, the activity of 5-α-reductase, and receptor affinity. Although there is no evidence of increased androgen production in men with acne, most women with acne do have increased ovarian androgen production and reduced SHBG concentrations. Undoubtedly, genetic factors also play an important part in determining which girls will suffer and which will not.

THE MENSTRUAL CYCLE

The menstrual cycle can be divided into two main stages which can be named from two different standpoints:
- The follicular and luteal phases – according to events in the ovary;
- The proliferative and secretory phases – according to changes that take place in the endometrium.

Since endometrial changes are dependent on the hormonal changes occurring in the ovary, the terms follicular phase and luteal phase will be used in this chapter.

FOLLICULAR PHASE

A few days before the onset of menstruation, the level of FSH starts to rise (**1.5**). This causes several antral follicles to start producing estradiol. As these follicles fill with fluid produced by the granulosa cells, which lie as a single layer around each follicle, they become visible on an ultrasound scan (**1.6**). In order to produce estradiol, the granulosa cells utilize

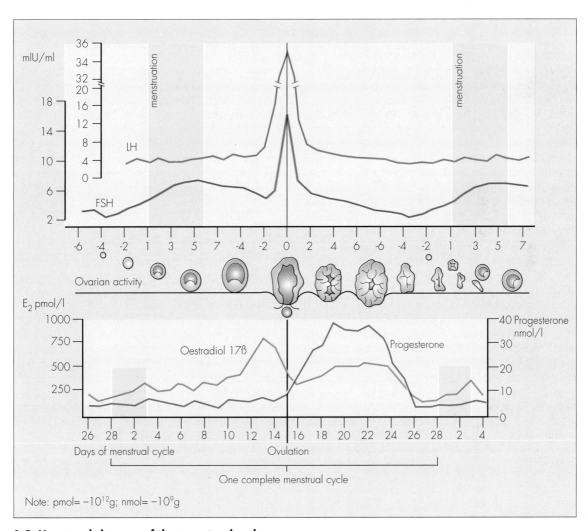

1.5 Hormonal changes of the menstrual cycle.

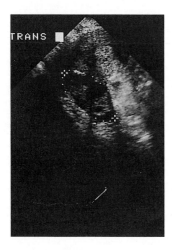

1.6 Early follicle. Transvaginal ultrasound scan of an early follicle (dia.8mm) in a normal ovary.

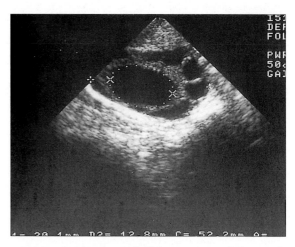

1.7 Mature dominant follicle. Transvaginal ultrasound scan of a mature dominant follicle (dia.18mm) in a polycystic ovary.

testosterone produced by the theca cells, which lie as a second monolayer around the follicle.

In the early follicular phase, the granulosa cells carry receptors for FSH, while the theca cells are stimulated by LH. The estradiol produced by the ovary is released into the circulation. The pituitary has an abundance of estradiol receptors – their activation results in the inhibition of both LH and FSH production in the mid-follicular phase. The granulosa cells also produce inhibin, a protein which augments the negative feedback of estradiol on FSH. This protein is also produced by the corpus luteum following ovulation. As a result of this effect, the smaller follicles stop growing and become atretic.

By this stage, only one follicle (but, occasionally, two or more) has reached a diameter of about 10–12mm, and is called the dominant follicle. The granulosa cells of the dominant follicle develop LH receptors and so become receptive to both LH and FSH. The follicle increases in diameter by 2mm per day. The estradiol concentrations rise faster and the granulosa cells begin to accumulate in several layers over the oocyte.

Oocyte Release

When the follicle reaches a diameter of around 18–20mm (**1.7**), and the estradiol concentration reaches 800–1000pmol/l, the biofeedback on the

pituitary is reversed. This results in a rapid rise in hormone concentrations, predominantly in LH and to a lesser extent in FSH.

In turn, this leads to a luteinization of the granulosa cells and consequently they begin to produce progesterone in preference to estradiol. This change leads to the rupture of the follicle wall, and the oocyte is released into the peritoneum about 24–36 hours after the LH surge. The follicular phase ends with release of the oocyte, and varies in length from 12 to16 days.

LUTEAL PHASE

This event marks the start of the luteal phase. Following release of the oocyte, the granulosa cells reseal the defect in the wall within a few hours, forming the corpus luteal cyst (**1.8**). The granulosa (now luteal) cells produce progesterone and this reaches a peak concentration 5–8 days after ovulation. The effect of progesterone on the endometrium is to increase the surface area of the endometrial glands and their blood supply by causing them to become spiral. They also start to produce large amounts of glycogen – an essential nutrient for the early days of embryo development if fertilization takes place.

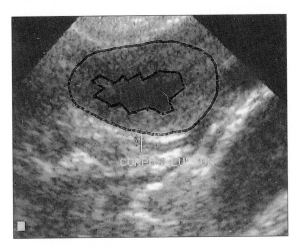

1.8 Corpus luteum. Transvaginal ultrasound scan of a corpus luteum in a normal ovary.

If the oocyte is fertilized and implantation occurs, then progesterone levels remain high. These levels are maintained by human chorionic gonadotrophin (hCG) produced by the trophoblastic elements of the embryo. If fertilization does not occur, then the LH concentrations are not sufficient to maintain production of progesterone by the corpus luteum. The concentrations decline and the endometrium becomes ischemic. Its superficial layers slough off. This, together with bleeding from the spiral arterioles which supplied the endometrium, produces menstruation.

Thus, the cycle has come full circle to the hormonal and endometrial states found at its beginning. The whole process then begins again.

SKIN CHANGES

Skin changes during the menstrual cycle are usually temporary and of minor importance. They include an increase in sebum production before menses, which may lead to acneiform eruptions on the face and occasionally on the back.

PREGNANCY

During the first few weeks of pregnancy, progesterone concentrations increase. Progesterone is initially produced by the corpus luteum, which is maintained by the production of human chorionic gonadotrophin (hCG) from the trophoblast of the conceptus.

Human chorionic gonadotrophin has been found in the maternal circulation almost immediately after fertilization and rises to a peak by 60–90 days of gestation. The concentration of hCG doubles every two or three days until this time, then gradually declines to a plateau level for the remainder of pregnancy.

The corpus luteum continues to produce progesterone, 17-hydroxyprogesterone, estrone, and estradiol, producing a rise in the concentration of all these hormones. In addition, hCG is responsible for the production of inhibin and relaxin by the corpus luteum.

Inhibin reduces FSH concentrations so that folliculogenesis is arrested once the embryo has become implanted into the endometrium. It may also act as a growth factor for the early embryo.

Relaxin is thought to act in synergy with progesterone to reduce the contractility of the uterine myometrium. The concentrations of both these hormones rise in parallel to the concentration of hCG, but they are produced for a limited period only by the ovary. From around seven weeks' gestation, they are produced by the decidual fetal membranes and placental tissues. Similarly, ovarian steroid hormone production declines from seven weeks' gestation, with the placental unit taking over this function. This explains why pregnancies will fail if the corpus luteum is removed before eight weeks, but will continue unharmed if the pregnancy has reached nine weeks' gestation.

THE PLACENTA

The placenta is a complex organ. Not only does it provide nutrients and excrete waste products from the fetus, but it also modifies the maternal metabolism at various stages of pregnancy via hormones. The placenta reaches structural maturity by the end of the 12th week of pregnancy. The functional unit is the chorionic villus which consists of a central core of

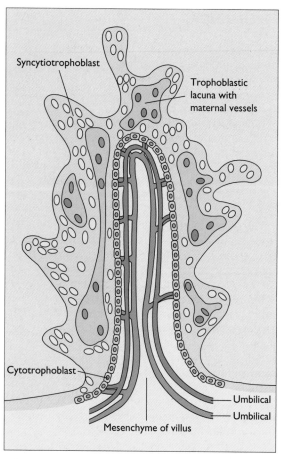

Syncytiotrophoblast

Trophoblastic lacuna with maternal vessels

Cytotrophoblast

Umbilical

Umbilical

Mesenchyme of villus

1.9 Chorionic villus. This shows the relationship of the cytotrophoblast with the syncytiotrophoblast and the fetal/maternal blood supply.

loose connective tissue and abundant capillaries. These connect to the fetal circulation, and provide a large surface area in contact with the maternal uterine circulation. Around this central core are two layers of trophoblast, an outer syncytium (syncytiotrophoblast), and an inner layer of discrete cells (cytotrophoblast) (**1.9**).

The fetus and the placenta form an interdependent partnership which regulates the endocrine–metabolic processes during pregnancy. This fetal–placental unit therefore becomes an endocrine system, producing a large number of different hormones (**Table 1.1**).

Several placental products have been measured over the years in the search for a marker for placental insufficiency. These include estriol and human placental lactogen (hPL), the concentrations of which rise steadily throughout pregnancy. But as their normal ranges are very large, they have not proved clinically useful in predicting the outcome of pregnancy.

Following the baby's birth, all the hormone levels return to normal within a few days. The production of hCG, progesterone, estriol, estradiol and hPL during pregnancy is shown in **1.10**. Despite our ability to measure these hormones during pregnancy, the role that they play in maintaining pregnancy and/or initiating parturition is still poorly understood.

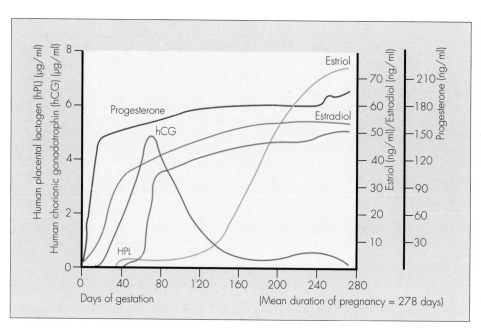

1.10 Hormonal changes during pregnancy. Changes in the production of progesterone, estradiol, estriol, human chorionic gonadotrophin, and human placental lactogen.

Peptides	Inhibin
	Relaxin
	Human placental lactogen
Neuropeptides	Gonadotrophin-releasing hormone
	Corticotrophin-releasing hormone
	Thyroid releasing hormone
Steroid hormones	Progesterone
	Androgens
	Estradiol
	Estrone
	Estriol
Peptide growth factors	Insulin-like growth factors I and II

Table 1.1. Hormones produced by the fetal–placental unit.

THE MENOPAUSE

The menopause marks the end of a woman's reproductive life. The average age for the end of menses in the UK is 50.3 years. During the years preceding the final cessation of menses, there is an increase in circulating FSH levels and a decrease in estradiol concentrations. The negative feedback of estradiol on FSH still occurs, but the resting concentration of FSH is higher than in younger women. The concentrations of FSH at the midcycle surge and in the late luteal phase are also greater. Luteinizing hormone levels tend to remain within the normal range until the cessation of menses. Raised concentrations of FSH are found in ovulatory cycles, providing evidence that the ovary gradually becomes less responsive to the gonadotrophins. The timing of menses may become more irregular, and many cycles are anovulatory, as the ovaries become depleted of antral follicles and no longer respond to FSH.

Estradiol levels gradually decline until they are so low that the endometrium no longer undergoes proliferation and becomes atrophic. The endometrium is no longer shed and menses cease. As well as a decline in estradiol levels, androgen levels also decrease from an average of 1.6nmol/l to 0.5nmol/l. This reduction in androgen levels has been used to explain the decrease in libido sometimes experienced by postmenopausal women.

As a secondary effect of reduced estradiol concentrations, FSH and LH levels rise owing to a lack of negative feedback on the pituitary gland. While the postmenopausal ovary produces minimal estradiol, it continues to produce quite significant amounts of testosterone and, to a lesser extent, androstenedione. These are presumably produced by the stromal cells of the ovary.

These androgens, predominantly adrenal androstenedione, are converted peripherally by aromatase into estrone. The extent to which this happens depends on age and weight. Heavier women have higher conversion rates and circulating estrogen concentrations than slim women. The average percentage of conversion in menopausal women is 2.8% and is double that found in premenopausal women. The relative change in balance between estrogen and androgen production in older women may account for the increased incidence of hirsutism in this group.

SKIN CHANGES

The skin changes in the vulva and vagina associated with the menopause seem to be secondary to low estradiol concentrations, since the topical application of estradiol can reverse them. Estradiol is essential to the maintenance of the elasticity and lubrication of the vagina.

The generalized aging process of the skin involves the vagina and vulva, as well as the rest of the body. The predominant process is progressive atrophy of the dermis and architectural changes leading to folds and wrinkles. The extent to which this occurs varies from individual to individual and depends on genetic and environmental factors.

In areas such as the vulva and vagina, which are protected from ultraviolet light, the epidermis becomes very thin. There is a reduced number of capillaries within the skin and elastotic changes occur in the arterioles. With time, the withdrawal of estrogens causes the vaginal skin to lose its folds, and the vaginal epithelium becomes thin and friable, making it more susceptible to trauma with the result that it bleeds. This is a very common cause of postmenopausal bleeding.

The atrophic changes that affect the vulva predispose it to trauma, often secondary to excessive itching. This may lead to ulceration or scar formation as the wounds heal. In a few women, this leads to fusion of the labia majora (**1.11, 1.12**).

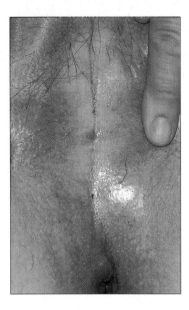

1.11 Fused labia. This condition has occurred secondary to postmenopausal skin changes.

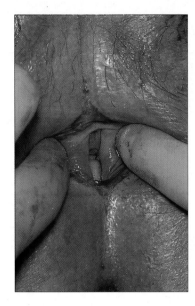

1.12 Surgical correction of fused labia. The same patient as in **1.11**, after surgical opening performed.

CONCLUSION

A woman's skin is affected by the many hormonal changes that occur during her lifetime. The degree to which each individual reacts depends on genetic and environmental factors. There is sound research to support the hormonal basis for some skin changes. However, the prevailing hormonal milieu is often used to provide a physiologic explanation for many other conditions that come and go – often regardless of changes in the woman's serum endocrinology. This is particularly true in pregnancy, and much work remains to be done to prove that current supposition is based on scientific fact.

REFERENCES

1 Gujeon, A. L. Rate of follicular growth in the human ovary. In: Rolland, R., van Hall, E. V., Hillier, S. G., *et al.* (eds.) Follicular maturation and ovulation. *Excerpta Medica*, Amsterdam, 1985, pp.155–163.

2 Apter, D., Bolton, N. J., and Hammond, G. L. Serum sex hormone binding globulin during puberty in girls and in different types of adolescent menstrual cycles. *Acta Endocrinol.* 1984; **107**: 413–419.

3 Cunningham, S. K., Loughlin, T., Culliton, M., *et al.* Plasma sex hormone binding globulin levels decline during the second decade of life irrespective of pubertal status. *J. Clin. Endocrinol. Metabol.* 1984; **58**: 915–918.

4 Smith, C. P., Archibald, H. R., Thomas, J. M., *et al.* Basal and stimulated insulin levels rise with advancing puberty. *Clin. Endocrinol.* 1988; **28**: 7–14.

5 Lawrence, D., Katz, M., Robinson, T. W., *et al.* Reduced sex hormone binding globulin and derived free testosterone levels in women with acne. *Clin. Endocrinol.* 1981; **15**: 87–91.

6 Burghen, G. A., Givens, J. R., and Kitabchi, A. E. Correlation of hyperandrogenism with hyperinsulinaemia in polycystic ovarian disease. *J. Clin. Endocrinol. Metabol.* 1980; **50**: 113–116.

7 Gollnick, H., Zoubilis, C., Akamatsu, H., *et al.* Pathogenesis and pathogenesis related treatment of acne. *J. Dermatol.* 1991; **18**: 489–499.

8 Pochi, P., Strauss, J., and Downing, D. Age-related changes in sebaceous gland activity. *J. Investig. Dermatol.* 1979; **73**: 108–111.

9 Simpson, N., Cunliffe, W., Rademaker, M., *et al.* The sebaceous gland as a source of androgen – an hypothesis. In: Marks, R. and Plewig, G. (eds.) *Acne and Related Disorders*. London: Martin Dunitz, 1989: p.27–30.

FURTHER READING

Yen, S. S. C. and Jaffe, R. B. (eds.) *Reproductive Endocrinology*. 3rd ed. Philadelphia: W. B. Saunders, 1991: Chapters 11, 25, 26.

2.
Perimenstrual Skin Eruptions; Autoimmune Progesterone Dermatitis

Catherine J. M. Stephens & Martin M. Black

Introduction

The activity of many skin diseases fluctuates in relation to the menstrual cycle. Some eruptions are confined to the premenstrual period and are considered as part of the premenstrual syndrome. Furthermore many chronic dermatoses also flare premenstrually. Since the menstrual cycle is controlled by the sex hormones, premenstrual deterioration is thought to be an effect of progesterone, the predominant circulating hormone of the premenstrual period. Hypersensitivity to progesterone can be demonstrated in a small number of these cases, when the condition is known as autoimmune progesterone dermatitis.

Sex Hormones and the Skin

The skin is highly sensitive to the effects of the sex steroid hormones, both to estrogen and progesterone, as well as to androgens.

Estrogens have been shown to suppress sebaceous activity but have little or no effect on the apocrine glands. They increase dermal hyaluronic acid levels with a consequent increase in the water content of the dermis and slow the breakdown of dermal collagen, possibly by increasing the conversion of soluble collagen to the insoluble form. Estrogens also stimulate epidermal melanogenesis, accounting for the transient hyperpigmentation that commonly occurs premenstrually, particularly around the eyes and nipples, and they have also been shown to slow the rate of hair growth. Estrogens alone appear to possess anti-inflammatory properties and will reduce the cutaneous response in delayed hypersensitivity reactions.

The way in which natural progesterone affects the skin is less clear. The vascularity of the skin is greatly increased during the second half of the menstrual cycle and there is increased sebaceous gland activity, producing seborrhea and, frequently, mild premenstrual acne. Although the mechanism of action is not known, these are both likely to be effects of progesterone.

The Perimenstrual Dermatoses

THE PREMENSTRUAL SYNDROME

Perimenstrual eruptions fall into three categories. An eruption recurring cyclically, and confined to the premenstrual period, may be considered part of the premenstrual syndrome (PMS) (**Table 2.1**).

A specific endocrine etiology for the PMS has not yet been defined. Changes in endorphins, prostaglandins and prolactin[1] have all been implicated, but because of the temporal association of symptoms with the luteal phase of the menstrual cycle, an abnormality of progesterone is strongly suspected[1]. Several hypotheses for a progesterone-related effect have been proposed, but not proven, including progesterone deficiency[2], a relative imbalance of estrogen and progesterone levels, and a progesterone allergy[3].

Acne vulgaris is the most common disorder treated by dermatologists. It is a disease of the pilosebaceous unit leading to the formation of open and closed comedones, papules, pustules, nodules, and cysts. The non-inflammatory lesions are open comedones (blackheads) and closed comedones (whiteheads). Papules and pustules constitute the superficial inflammatory lesions, and cysts and nodules and occasionally deep pustules make up the deep lesions. In most patients several types of acne lesions are present simultaneously. In *mild acne,* scattered comedones and/or papules with a few pustules predominate. In *moderate acne* more papules and pustules are present (**2.2**), whereas

Seborrhea, acne vulgaris
Edema, weight gain
Nausea, vomiting
Constipation, frequency of micturition
Breast fullness/tenderness
Headache, migraine
Excitability, irritability
Lethargy, malaise, depression

Table 2.1   The Premenstrual Syndrome.

nodular–cystic lesions usually predominate in *severe acne*.

Mild facial acne is reported by up to 70% of women during the premenstrual period, often accompanied by excessive greasiness of the scalp. Perioral dermatitis, which is common in teenage girls, is quite frequently cyclical. In addition, edema of the hands and feet and more rarely patchy pigmentation of the skin may occur transiently as part of the premenstrual syndrome.

If premenstrual acne requires treatment, a topical antiseptic/keratolytic preparation (e.g. benzoyl peroxide) or antibiotic (e.g. clindamycin 1% solution) is usually helpful, but suppression of ovulation, and thus the post-ovulatory surge of progesterone, can also be effective. The choice of oral contraceptive pill is also important, as some synthetic progestogens, e.g. norethisterone and levonorgestrel, tend to make acne worse (**2.1**). For any acne-prone patient, a combined pill containing gestodene, desogestrel, or norgestimate is recommended. These progestogens appear not to have a stimulatory effect on sebaceous glands. Conversely, they raise levels of sex hormone-binding globulin, so reducing free testosterone, producing a clinical anti-androgenic effect[4].

Although a progestogen is frequently prescribed for symptoms of the premenstrual syndrome in which a functional deficit of natural progesterone is suspected[2] it currently has no place in the management of premenstrual acne.

PREMENSTRUAL EXACERBATION OF EXISTING DERMATOSES

Many women complain of cyclical premenstrual worsening of existing dermatoses (**Table 2.2**). This is a common phenomenon. Inflammatory disorders,

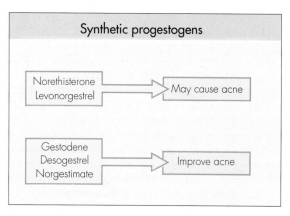

2.1 Synthetic progestogens used in the combined oral contraceptive pill which may affect acne.

| Acne vulgaris |
| Acne rosacea |
| Lupus erythematosus |
| Psoriasis |
| Atopic eczema |
| Lichen planus |
| Dermatitis herpetiformis |
| Pompholyx |
| Urticaria |
| Erythema multiforme |
| Pruritus vulvae |
| Pemphigoid gestationis |

Table 2.2 Chronic dermatoses that may flare premenstrually.

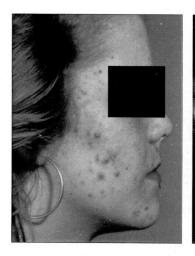
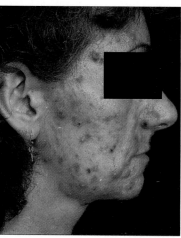

2.2 Acne vulgaris. Premenstrual flares are extremely common. Mild (**left**); severe (**right**).

particularly of the face, become more active and irritable premenstrually, in part due to the hormonal effects of increased cutaneous vascularity, seborrhea, and dermal edema. Acne vulgaris (**2.2**), rosacea (**2.3**), and the various forms of lupus erythematosus (**2.4**) are notable examples. Premenstrual flares are also well recognized in young women with psoriasis, atopic eczema (**2.5**), lichen planus, dermatitis herpetiformis[5], pompholyx, and urticaria. Pemphigoid gestationis may persist postpartum, classically falling into a pattern of premenstrual exacerbations[6]. Herpes simplex and aphthosis, although frequently recurrent, are often not strictly cyclical.

Increased cutaneous vascularity and the increased metabolic rate that occurs premenstrually will aggravate pruritic conditions, e.g. eczema and pruritus vulvae, and in general, tolerance of a dermatosis will often be lowered in women with premenstrual tension at this time of the cycle.

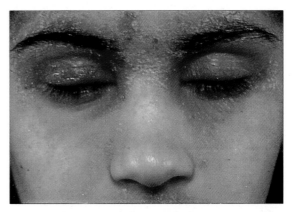

2.5 Atopic eczema is frequently less manageable premenstrually. Here, the dermatitis involves the eyelids as well as more typical areas such as the antecubital and popliteal fossae.

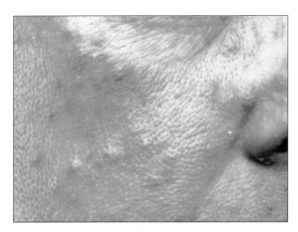

2.3 Acne rosacea may flare premenstrually.

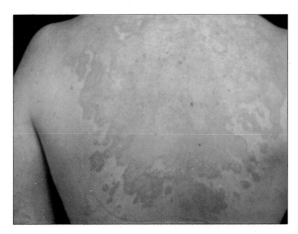

2.4 Subacute cutaneous lupus erythematosus.

AUTOIMMUNE PROGESTERONE DERMATITIS

Autoimmune progesterone dermatitis (AIPD) is a very rare condition characterized by recurrent premenstrual exacerbations of a dermatosis in which sensitivity to progesterone can be demonstrated.

History

The first case report of a cyclical eruption in which an allergy to endogenous sex hormones was suggested was by Geber[7], who in 1921 reported a case of menstrual urticaria in which the eruption could be reproduced by autoinjection of premenstrual serum. The concept of sex hormone sensitization was extended in 1945 when Zondek and Bromberg[8] described several patients with conditions related to menstruation and the menopause, including cases of cyclical urticaria. They demonstrated positive delayed hypersensitivity reactions to intradermal progesterone in affected patients but not in healthy controls, evidence of passive cutaneous transfer of skin reagins, and clinical suppression by desensitization.

In 1951, Guy[9] reported a case of premenstrual urticaria which reacted strongly to intradermal injections of extracts of corpus luteum and was later successfully treated by desensitization. The term autoimmune progesterone dermatitis was eventually introduced in 1964 by Shelley *et al.*[10] who were also the first to document a partial response to estrogens, and cure by oophorectomy.

Clinical Manifestations

Twenty-eight cases of AIPD have been reported to date in the English literature. Various clinical morphological features are described including eczema (**2.6**)[11–13], erythema multiforme (**2.7, 2.8**)[10,13–16], urticaria (**2.9**)[9,13,17–19], pompholyx [13,20], stomatitis[21], and a dermatitis herpetiformis-like eruption (**2.10**)[5] (**Table 2.3**). The eruptions do not appear to differ morphologically or histologically from the non-cyclical variants. The condition is confined to ovulating women. Onset is usually in early adult life, occasionally after a normal pregnancy, and the duration is very variable, with spontaneous remissions occurring. Two-thirds of cases have been exposed to exogenous progesterone in the form of the oral contraceptive pill prior to the eruption[13,22]. Typically the dermatosis appears to flare during the second half of the menstrual cycle, peaks premenstrually and regresses spontaneously with the menstrual flow. Skin lesions are less florid, or the skin may be clear during the first

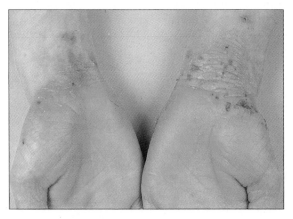

2.6 Autoimmune progesterone dermatitis. Flexural lichenified eczema.

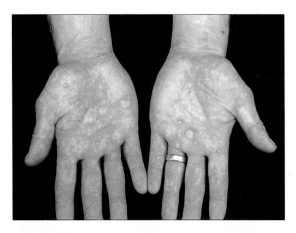

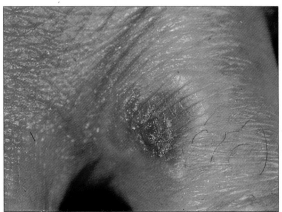

2.7, 2.8 Autoimmune progesterone dermatitis. Erythema multiforme.

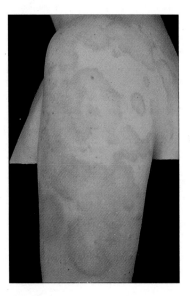

2.9 Auto-immune progesterone dermatitis. Polycyclic urticarial lesions.

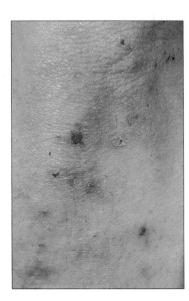

2.10 Auto-immune progesterone dermatitis. Excoriated papules over the elbows resembling dermatitis herpetiformis.

Eczema
Erythema multiforme
Urticaria
Pompholyx
Stomatitis
Dermatitis herpetiformis
Non-specific papular erythema

Table 2.3 Autoimmune Progesterone Dermatitis.

half of the cycle. By definition the eruption clinically recurs during every ovulatory cycle.

Mechanism of Sensitization

The mechanism by which women become sensitive to their own progesterone is not known. One frequently quoted hypothesis is that previous use of exogenous progestogens induces allergy to endogenous progesterone. It is suggested that synthetic progesterone is sufficiently antigenic to act as a stimulus for antibodies which then cross-react with natural progesterone and perpetuate the immune response premenstrually[13]. However, not all women with AIPD have been exposed to synthetic progestogens. Schoenmakers *et al.*[23] suggested that steroid cross-sensitivity could be an alternative sensitizing mechanism after demonstrating cross-sensitivity on cutaneous testing between hydrocortisone and 17-hydroxyprogesterone in five of 19 corticosteroid-sensitive women, two of whom had features of AIPD. We were, however, unable to demonstrate steroid cross-sensitivity in five of our patients with AIPD and obtained no positive reactions to 17-hydroxyprogesterone[24].

Pregnancy

Three cases report onset or a worsening of the eruption during pregnancy[16,25,26], as well as premenstrual exacerbations. This is not unexpected, as progesterone and estrogen levels rise steadily throughout pregnancy. Two cases were associated with spontaneous abortion. However, spontaneous improvement or clearing during pregnancy is reported in other cases[11,17,18].

Pregnancy is known to ameliorate many allergic states; therefore it is suggested that there is a low maternal immunological reaction during pregnancy, probably due to the elevated cortisol levels that occur. One could also postulate that the gradual rise in the hormone levels during pregnancy brings about hormonal desensitization in some individuals.

EVIDENCE FOR PROGESTERONE SENSITIVITY

All cases of AIPD show cyclical premenstrual exacerbations of the eruption (**2.11**), which, with the use of accurate diary cards, may be shown to correspond to the post-ovulation rise in serum progesterone. In addition, the eruption is frequently resistant to conventional therapy, irrespective of clinical type, but responds to anovulatory drugs. This implies sex hormone sensitivity, but not necessarily an antibody-mediated reaction to progesterone.

Hypersensitivity to progesterone may be demonstrated by controlled intradermal tests, intramuscular or oral progesterone challenge, or the demonstration of circulating antibodies to progesterone[12,27] or the corpus luteum [17,27]. Two cases have been associated with a serum binding factor to 17-hydroxyprogesterone[28,29].

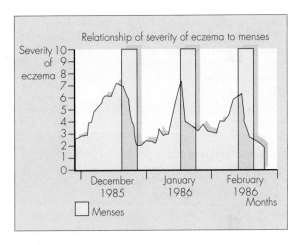

2.11 Autoimmune progesterone dermatitis.
Patients' diary cards confirms recurrent premenstrual exacerbations of eczema.

Progesterone Intradermal Tests

Intradermal tests using synthetic progesterone are reported to show an immediate positive urticarial reaction in some cases, but more frequently a delayed hypersensitivity reaction. Intradermal tests, although frequently used, in our experience are unpredictable because of the insolubility of progesterone in water, and the fact that all diluents are highly irritant. Reactions are often difficult to interpret, and false positive reactions can occur (**2.12**). Furthermore, skin necrosis at test sites producing scarring often occurs (**2.13**). However, a persistent late reaction confined to test sites implies progesterone sensitivity.

Recommended Procedures for Progesterone Intradermal Tests

Various dilutions of progesterone solution 0.2ml, plus controls of diluent alone are injected intradermally into the anterior aspect of the forearm to produce a well-defined raised bleb. Pure progesterone powder is solubilized using a 60% ethanol/saline mixture to produce 1%, 0.1% and 0.01% test solutions. Ethanol/saline (60%) alone and normal saline should be used as controls. Estrogen sensitivity may be investigated concurrently using ethinylestradiol and the same diluent. Readings should be made every 10 minutes for half-an-hour then every 30 minutes for the first four hours and at 24 and 48 hours. Immediate irritant reactions to diluent alone may occur, in which case all early reactions at test sites should be discounted.

A positive reaction to progesterone is said to occur if a persistent wheal and flare reaction is present exclusively at the progesterone test sites, between 24 and 48 hours (**2.14**).

Intramuscular and Oral Progesterone Challenge

Challenge with intramuscular progesterone has been reported in six cases and produced a flare of the eruption in all six patients. Testing should be undertaken during the first half of the menstrual cycle when the eruption would normally be quiescent, and the patient observed carefully as severe exacerbations of urticaria with angioedema, although extremely uncommon, have been reported. We have used Gestone (Paines & Byrne), 25mg/ml, successfully for intramuscular challenge.

Placebo-controlled oral challenge may also be of value, again if performed during the first half of the menstrual cycle. Dydrogesterone 10mg daily for seven days or levonorgestrel 30µg made up to 500mg capsules with lactose, one per day for seven days followed by seven days of lactose-only capsules may be used. Oral challenge is less reliable, as the eruption may not flare dramatically and may therefore be difficult to interpret.

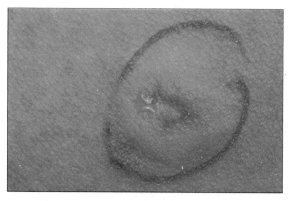

2.13 Autoimmune progesterone dermatitis. Skin necrosis at sites of progesterone intradermal tests commonly occurs.

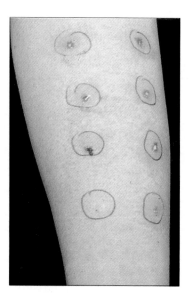

2.12 Progesterone intradermal testing demonstrating irritant reactions with necrosis at test sites. Such results cannot be interpreted.

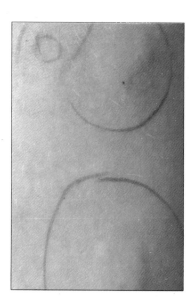

2.14 Positive progesterone intradermal tests. Persistent wheal and flare at two progesterone test sites.

Challenge Following Chemical Oophorectomy

The optimum test for AIPD, only to be recommended if the patient is so severely affected as to be considering surgical oophorectomy, is to perform a chemical oophorectomy using subcutaneous injections of an LHRH antagonist over a six-month period, and document clearance of the eruption alongside hormonal confirmation of absence of ovulation. Goserelin 3.6mg by subcutaneous injection may be used for this purpose. If progesterone challenge then produces a flare of the eruption, this is substantial evidence for progesterone sensitivity.

TREATMENT

The majority of cases of AIPD encountered have failed to respond to conventional treatment modalities, although oral prednisone (prednisolone) in moderately high doses may bring about control[11,15,20]. Many cases, however, respond well to conjugated estrogens, presumably by suppression of ovulation and hence the post-ovulatory rise in progesterone. In practice, however, estrogen therapy is often not appropriate in view of the usual patients' age. When estrogen therapy is unsuccessful, the antiestrogen/anovulatory drug tamoxifen may be tried. Tamoxifen 30mg has caused complete remission in three patients[11,16,24] but with consequent amenorrhea. A lower dose was achieved in one patient with return of menstruation but not the rash. No side effects were encountered.

In severe cases, oophorectomy will clear the eruption. Surgical oophorectomy has cured one patient[10], and suppression of AIPD urticaria by chemical oophorectomy using the LHRH analogue Buserilin has been reported[30].

In our experience many cases of AIPD slowly settle spontaneously after a period of successful treatment.

REFERENCES

1 Strickler, R.C. Endocrine hypothesis for the aetiology of premenstrual syndrome. *Clin. Obstet. Gynaecol.* 1987; **30**: 377–383.

2 Dalton, K. *The Premenstrual Syndrome and Progesterone Therapy.* 2nd Ed. Chicago: Year Book Medical Publishers 1984.

3 Maxson WS. The use of progesterone in the treatment of PMS. *Clin. Obstet. Gynaecol.* 1987; **30**: 465–477.

4 *Drug and Therapeutic Bulletin* 1992; **30**: 41–44.

5 Leitao, E.A.and Bernhard, J.D. Perimenstrual nonvascular dermatitis herpetiformis. *J. Amer. Acad. Dermatol.* 1990; **22**: 331–334.

6 Holmes, .Black, M.M. The specific dermatoses of pregnancy – a reappraisal with specific emphasis on a proposal simplified clinical classification. *Clin. Exp. Dermatol.* 1982; **7**: 65–73.

7 Geber, H. Einege daten zur pathologie dur urticaria menstruationalis. *Dermatol. Z.* 1921; **32**: 143–150.

8 Zondek, B. and Bromberg, Y.M. Endocrine allergy: allergic sensitivity to endogenous hormones. *J. Allergy* 1945; **16**: 1–16.

9 Guy, W.H., Jacobs, F.M. and Guy, W.B. Sex hormone sensitisation (corpus luteum). *Arch. Dermatol.* 1951; **63**: 377–378.

10 Shelley, W.B., Prencel, R.W.and Spoont, S.S. Autoimmune progesterone dermatitis: cure by oophorectomy. *JAMA* 1964; **190**: 35–38.

11 Stephens, C.J.M., Wojnarowska, F.T. and Wilkinson, J.D. Autoimmune progesterone dermatitis responding to tamoxifen. *Br. J. Dermatol.* 1989; **121**: 135–137.

12 Jones, W.N.and Gordon, V.H. Autoimmune progesterone eczema: an endogenous progesterone hypersensitivity. *Arch. Dermatol.* 1969; **99**: 57–59.

13 Hart, R. Autoimmune progesterone dermatitis. *Arch. Dermatol.* 1977; **113**: 426–430.

14 Stone, J.and Downham, T. Autoimmune progesterone dermatitis. *Int. J. Dermatol.* 1981; **20**: 50–51.

15 Torras, H., Fenaudo, H.and Mallolas, J. Dermatitis postovulation. *Med. Cutan. Ibero Lat. Am.* 1980; **8**: 15–22.

16 Wojnarowska, F., Greaves, M.W.and Peachey, R.D. Progesterone induced erythema multiforme. *J. R. Soc. Med.* 1985; **78**: 407–408.

17 Farah, F.S.and Shbaklu, Z. Autoimmune progesterone urticaria. *J. Allergy Clin. Immunol.* 1971; **48**: 357–361.

18 Georgouras, K. Autoimmune progesterone dermatitis. *Aust. J. Dermatol.* 1981; **22**: 109–111.

19 Tromovitch, T.and Heggli, W. Autoimmune progesterone urticaria. *Calif. Med.* 1967; **106**: 211–212.

20 Anderson, R.H. Autoimmune progesterone dermatitis. *Cutis* 1984; **33**: 490–491.

21 Berger, H. Ulcerative stomatitis caused by endogenous progesterone. *Ann. Intern. Med.* 1955; **42**: 205–208.

22 Stephens, C.J.M.and Black, M.M. Perimenstrual eruptions: autoimmune progesterone dermatitis. *Semin. Dermatol.* 1989; **8**: 26–29.

23 Schoenmakers, A., Vermorken, A., Degreef, H.and Dooms-Goossens, A. Corticosteroid or steroid allergy?. *Contact Dermatitis.* 1992: **26** 159–162.

24 Stephens, C.J.M., McFadden, J.P., Black, M.M.B.and Rycroft, R.J.G. Autoimmune progesterone dermatitis. Absence of contact sensitivity to glucocorticoids, oestrogen and 17-OH-Progesterone (In press).

25 Mayou, S.C., Charles-Holmes, R., Kenney, A.and Black, M.M. A Premenstrual eruption treated with bilateral oophorectomy and hysterectomy. *Clin. Exp. Dermatol.* 1988; **13**: 114–116.

26 Bierman, S.M. Autoimmune progesterone dermatitis of pregnancy. *Arch. Dermatol.* 1973; **107**: 896–961.

27 Veda, T., Matuda, M.and Yambe, H. *et al.* Two cases of autoimmune progesterone dermatitis, in Wilkinson, D.S., Mascaro, J.M.and Orfanes, C.E. (eds). *Clinical Dermatology. The CMD Case Collection.* New York, Schattauer Stuggart 1987; 214–215.

28 Pinto, J.S., Sobrinho, L., da Silva, M.B., Porto, M.T., Santos, M.A., Balo-Banga, M.AND Arala-Chaves, M. Erythema multiforme associated with autoreactivity to 17 hydroxyprogesterone. *Dermatologica* 1990; **26**: 159–162.

29 Cheesman, K.L., Gaynor, L.V., Chatterton, R.T., Jr.,and Radvany, R.M. Identification of a 17-hydroxyprogesterone-binding immunoglobulin in the serum of a woman with periodic rashes. *J. Clin. Endocrinol. Metabol.* 1982; **55**: 597–599.

30 Yee, K.C. and Cunliffe, W.J. Progesterone-induced urticaria: response to buserilin. *Brit. J. Dermatol.* 1994; **130**: 121–123.

3.
Physiologic Changes of Pregnancy

Marilynne McKay

HYPERPIGMENTATION

Localized or generalized hyperpigmentation occurs to some extent in 90% of pregnant women. These changes are most prominent in patients with darkly pigmented skin, although they occur to some degree in fair-skinned individuals. Perhaps the most familiar example is the darkening of the linea alba. This is described in obstetrical textbooks as an early change of pregnancy, but it may not be apparent until several months gestation, especially in a first pregnancy. The midline streak usually proceeds from the symphysis pubis to the umbilicus, but can extend to the xiphoid process (**3.1–3.4**). It tends to appear earlier in subsequent pregnancies.

The nipples and aureolae become pigmented (**3.2–3.4**), as do the external genitalia and the axillae

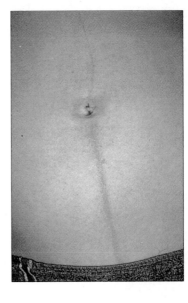

3.1 Hyper-pigmentation. Darkening of the linea alba from the symphysis pubis to the xiphoid process during pregnancy.

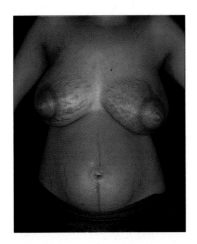 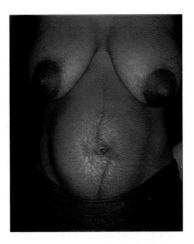 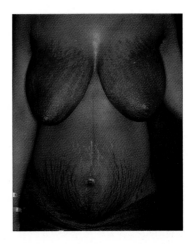

3.2–3.4 Hyperpigmentation. Three different patterns of skin darkening in African-Americans, as seen immediately postpartum. Note the differences in striae formation on the abdomen and breasts, as well as patterns of pigmentation of the linea nigra, nipples, and aureolae.

(**3.5**). Darkening of the neck is particularly bothersome to some patients (**3.6**), but this gradually fades postpartum, along with any other pigmentary changes. Striae ('stretch marks') are common, and may darken in susceptible individuals (**3.7**), along with other scars, nevi, and freckles. Vulvar melanosis may also develop during pregnancy (**3.8**).

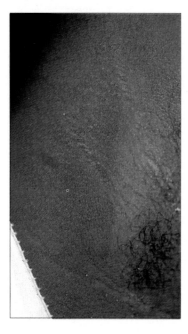

3.5 Hyperpigmentation. Pseudoacanthotic pigmentation of the axilla in another African-American, who also had darkening of the vulva.

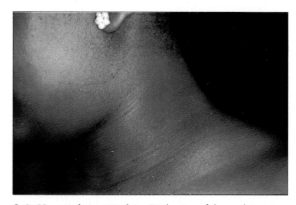

3.6 Hyperpigmentation. Darkening of the neck in an African-American. This is cosmetically distressing to some patients, but will fade slowly.

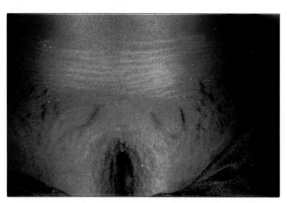

3.7 Striae distensae. Pigmentation of new striae which have developed during pregnancy; older striae remain pale.

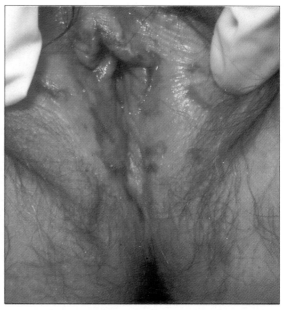

3.8 Vulvar melanosis. This benign change developed during pregnancy and did not require treatment.

PIGMENTARY DEMARCATION LINES

Some dark-skinned people (male and female) have pigmentary demarcation lines (also called Voight's or Futcher's lines) along the outer portion of the upper arms and/or posterior legs. These may not have been noticed by the patient until the general darkening of pigment during pregnancy makes them more prominent (**3.9,3.10**).

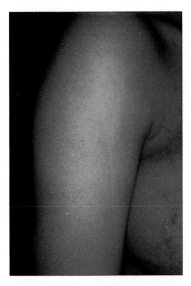

3.9 Pigmentary demarction line. This can be seen on the upper arm. It has become more prominent during pregnancy.

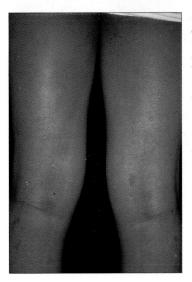

3.10 Pigmentary demarcation lines. These lines, also known as Voight's or Futcher's lines, can be seen on the posterior legs. They were not noticed by the patient until they darkened during pregnancy.

MELASMA

Melasma (formerly called chloasma, or the 'mask of pregnancy') is macular hyperpigmentation of the face (**3.11**). Although the malar pattern is considered typical, the entire central face is affected in most patients, including the forehead, cheeks, upper lip, nose, and chin. It occurs in the second trimester in three-fourths of pregnant women and one-third of those on oral contraceptive pills (OCPs). It is thought to be due to hormonal influences, and is worsened by sun exposure. It usually fades within a year after pregnancy or discontinuation of OCPs.

Melasma is persistent in approximately 30% of patients, whether induced by pregnancy or estrogen-containing OCPs. Epidermal pigment (accentuated by Woods light examination) is most responsive to bleaching with topical hydroquinone creams and tretinoin.

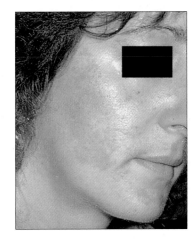

3.11 Melasma. The 'mask of pregnancy' in a typical distribution on the central face.

STRIAE DISTENSAE

The so-called 'stretch marks', which occur in almost all pregnant women during the second and third trimester, are linear, pink-to-purplish, atrophic lines that develop at right angles to the skin tension lines on the abdomen, breasts, buttocks, thighs, and groin

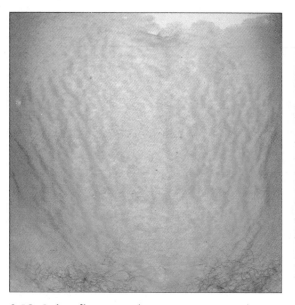

3.12 Striae distensae. These are striae, or 'stretch marks' over a fair-skinned abdomen.

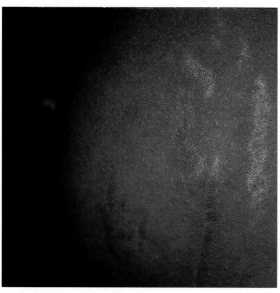

3.13 Striae distensae. Non-pigmented striae in an African-American.

(**3.12,3.13**). They are the same as those seen with Cushing's syndrome, steroid therapy, and rapid changes in body weight. The red coloration typically becomes flesh-colored or pale with time (with or without topical creams of various kinds), but although the atrophic lines may be thinner after delivery, they do not disappear completely. Topical tretinoin, 0.1% cream, has recently been shown to improve the appearance of striae.

HAIR AND NAIL CHANGES

Hirsutism – profuse growth of body hair – is seen in most pregnant women. It is more noticeable in women with dark and/or abundant body hair. The short lanugo hairs give the skin a 'furry' appearance; however, these disappear postpartum with the development of telogen effluvium.

Telogen effluvium results in the loss of terminal scalp hairs about one to five months postpartum – this hair loss can last up to a year or more before regrowth occurs (**3.14**). The best explanation for this phenomenon is that pregnancy interrupts the normal hair-shedding cycle, so allowing hairs to keep growing until delivery. Following delivery, the hair follicles rapidly resume their normal pattern of hair loss and regrowth, resulting in an apparently excessive loss of hair. However, patients can be reassured that baldness will not be the result.

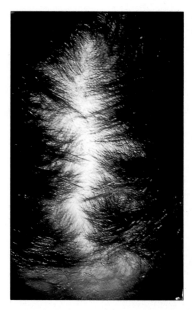

3.14 Telogen effluvium.

In rare cases, male-pattern baldness or diffuse thinning of scalp hairs may be seen late in pregnancy, but this also reverts to a normal pattern of hair growth postpartum.

Nail changes usually begin in the first trimester. Brittleness or softening may be seen, as can faster growth. Transverse grooving (Beau's line) has been noted after delivery, but this is a very nonspecific finding.

MUCOUS MEMBRANE CHANGES

Gingivitis of pregnancy is common, and occurs to greater or lesser degrees in most women. Hypertrophy of the gums increases gradually throughout pregnancy, and the mucosa become red and friable. Pyogenic granuloma (granuloma gravidarum) may be seen in this setting, but lesions usually regress after delivery and no treatment is required. They are thought to be caused by trauma to inflamed mucosa (**3.15, 3.16**).

VASCULAR AND HEMATOLOGIC CHANGES

Varicosities occur to some extent in almost half of all pregnancies, and are particularly bothersome around the anus (hemorrhoids) and on the legs (**3.17**). Leg and ankle edema is common and may also be accompanied by swelling of the hands and eyelids. For varicosities and swelling of the legs, supportive care with leg elevation and elastic stockings is recommended. Patients should avoid prolonged standing or sitting.

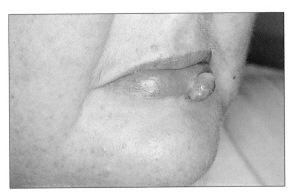

3.15 Pyogenic granuloma on the lip.

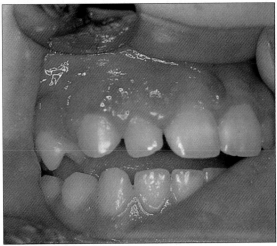

3.16 Pyogenic granuloma on the gingiva.

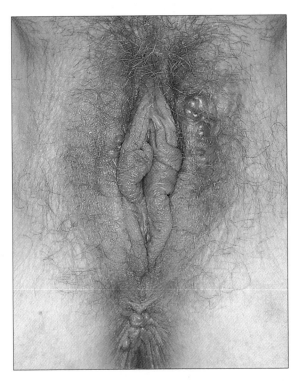

3.17 Hemorrhoids and vulvar varicosities developing during pregnancy.

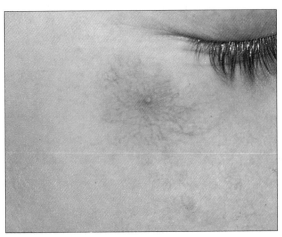

3.18 Vascular spider.

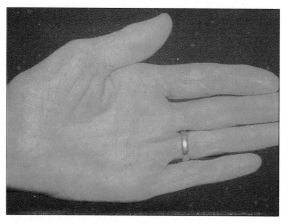

3.19 Palmar erythema.

Spider angiomas (nevus araneus, spider nevus) usually develop in the first and second trimesters. Easily recognized by a central red punctum with radiating branches on the upper body, they may be seen in two-thirds of pregnant white women (**3.18**). Palmar erythema is also common in about the same number of patients (**3.19**). The etiology of both is unknown, but is thought to be associated with estrogen or angiogenic factors. These changes usually resolve postpartum.

FURTHER READING

Callen, J. P. Pregnancy's effects on the skin: common and uncommon changes. *Postgrad. Med.* 1984; **75**: 138–145.

Elson, M. L. Treatment of striae distensae with topical tretinoin. *J. Dermatol. Surg. Oncol.* 1990; **16**: 267–270.

James, W. D., Guill, M. A., Berger, T. G., *et al.* Pigmentary demarcation lines associated with pregnancy. *J. Am. Acad. Dermatol.* 1984; **11**: 438–440.

Martin, A. G. and Leal-Khouri, S. Physiologic skin changes associated with pregnancy. *Int. J. Dermatol.* 1992; **31**: 375–378.

Wong, R. C. and Ellis, C. N. Physiologic skin changes in pregnancy. *J. Am. Acad. Dermatol.* 1984; **10**: 929–940.

Wong, R. C. and Ellis, C. N. Physiologic skin changes in pregnancy. *Semin. Dermatol.* 1989; **8**: 7–11.

Winton, G. B. and Lewis, C. W. Dermatoses of pregnancy. *J. Am. Acad. Dermatol.* 1982; **6**: 977–998.

Wade, T. R., Wade, S. L., and Jones, H. E. Skin changes and diseases associated with pregnancy. *Obstet. Gynecol.* 1978; **52**: 233–242.

ACKNOWLEDGEMENTS

Figures **3.1** and **3.11** are reproduced from C.M. Lawrence and N.H. Cox *Color Atlas and Text of Physical Signs in Dermatology* (Figs 6.28 and 6.27), Wolfe, London 1993. Figure **3 12** is reproduced from G.M. Levene and C.D. Calnan *Color Atlas of Dermatology* (Fig 464), Mosby–Wolfe, London1994. Figure **3.16** is reproduced from W.R. Tyldesley *Color Atlas of Oral Medicine* (Fig 146), Mosby–Wolfe, London 1994. Figure **3.19** is reproduced from V.R. Tindall *Diagnostic Picture Tests in Obstetrics and Gynaecology* (Fig 91), Wolfe, London 1987.

4.
A Systematic Approach to the Dermatoses of Pregnancy

Martin M. Black

INTRODUCTION

Cutaneous symptoms and signs are not uncommon during pregnancy. The physiologic signs of pregnancy (*see also Chapter 3*) often involve the skin or mucous membranes, and can sometimes provide contributory evidence of pregnancy.

Although pruritus is the principal cutaneous symptom in pregnancy, itching in itself is not diagnostically helpful. Thus, a full clinical history and a thorough clinical examination are essential to confirm, or exclude, the possibility of any coexisting dermatosis or infestation. The clinical implications of pruritus in pregnancy are outlined in **Table 4.1.**

Chapter 8 describes the effect of pregnancy on other skin disorders. This chapter will deal with pruritus gravidarum and the difficult nomenclature of the specific dermatoses of pregnancy.

Normal skin (pruritus gravidarum)
Cholestasis of pregnancy
Associated skin rash
Pre-existing skin condition
Coincidentally acquired skin condition
Specific dermatosis of pregnancy

Table 4.1 Clinical Implications of Pruritus in Pregnancy.

INTRAHEPATIC CHOLESTASIS OF PREGNANCY (PRURITUS GRAVIDARUM)

Intrahepatic cholestasis of pregnancy (ICP) is manifested by pruritus in pregnancy, with or without laboratory evidence of cholestasis[1]. Although the condition is not accompanied by primary skin lesions, excoriations due to severe scratching are often present in more severe cases[2].

The disorder is a genetically linked, estrogen-dependent condition, which results in cholestasis, with or without jaundice. It usually begins in later pregnancy and resolves rapidly after delivery[1,2,3,4]. A diagnosis of ICP can be readily established or confirmed using the criteria given in **Table 4.2.**

Pruritus related to pregnancy, with no history of exposure to hepatitis or hepatotoxic drugs
Presence of generalized pruritus with or without jaundice
Alteration of liver function tests consistent with cholestasis
Rapid disappearance of itching after delivery
Recurrence of itching in any subsequent pregnancy

Table 4.2 Diagnostic Criteria of Intrahepatic Cholestasis of Pregnancy.

PATHOGENESIS

No single biochemical abnormality has been found in ICP. It has been postulated that the relative fall in hepatic blood flow during pregnancy leads to decreased clearance of toxins, and also estrogens[5]. Estrogens increase biliary cholesterol concentration and secretion, and also impair the capacity of the liver to transport anions, such as bilirubin and bile salts.

It has also been postulated that estrogens regulate actin molecules, which act intracellularly to mediate bile excretion[6].

CLINICAL AND LABORATORY FINDINGS

The disorder typically presents in the last trimester of an otherwise normal pregnancy, but it can occasionally develop much earlier. Intense, generalized itching occurs, which is invariably worse at night, and persists throughout the duration of pregnancy. The result of physical examination is usually normal, apart from the finding of widespread excoriations.

About 50% of cases will develop darker urine and light-colored stools, but only a few will develop jaundice, usually within 2–4 weeks of the onset of itching.

A typical biochemical finding is of markedly increased serum bile acids. Other laboratory findings may include moderately increased levels of serum-conjugated bilirubin, alkaline phosphatase, cholesterol, and lipids. Liver transaminases are usually only slightly elevated; significantly higher levels of transaminases indicate that infectious hepatitis is the likely cause of the jaundice. Hepatic ultrasonographic findings are normal and liver biopsy is not indicated for typical ICP.

JAUNDICE

The incidence of jaundice in pregnancy is about 1 in every 1500 pregnancies[5]. For comparison, viral hepatitis is a more common cause of jaundice in pregnancy. Meanwhile, ICP accounts for about 20% of cases of obstetric jaundice. Since there is often a family history of obstetric jaundice, a possible genetic enzyme defect might be responsible.

FETAL RISKS

Intrahepatic cholestasis of pregnancy is associated with a high incidence of stillbirth and perinatal complications[7,8]. Intensive fetal surveillance is therefore recommended, including amniocentesis for meconium[6,7]. Induction at 38 weeks' gestation, or after demonstration of a mature lecithin to sphingomyelin ratio, may result in increased fetal survival[7,8].

MANAGEMENT

Treatment of the mother is largely symptomatic[1]. Cholestyramine or phenobarbital can be given, but there is no consensus about their efficacy. Phototherapy using ultraviolet B radiation may help relieve pruritus. In prolonged ICP, intramuscular administration of vitamin K may be necessary.

THE SPECIFIC DERMATOSES OF PREGNANCY

A group of inflammatory dermatoses closely related to pregnancy have caused great diagnostic confusion. Prior to 1982, the terminology became increasingly confused, with several names being used for similar clinical conditions (**Tables 4.3 and 4.4**). The author has extensively reviewed all the existing literature and has comprehensively studied a large group of patients, covering all the existing disease entities. Similar work was done by Holmes *et al.* before they published their proposals in 1982[19] and 1983[20] of a simplified, clinical classification of the specific dermatoses of pregnancy. This classification basically subdivided the specific dermatoses of pregnancy into four groups:
- Pemphigoid (herpes) gestationis;
- Polymorphic eruption of pregnancy;
- Prurigo of pregnancy;
- Pruritic folliculitis of pregnancy.

Unfortunately, except for pemphigoid (herpes) gestationis, no reliable criteria exist to differentiate the specific dermatoses of pregnancy[21]. Nevertheless, the proposed, simplified, clinical classification appears to have gradually gained international acceptance[21]. For example, a recent prospective study of

Disorder	Original Author(s)	Date
Herpes gestationis	Milton[9]	1872
Herpes impetiginiformis (impetigo herpetiformis)	Hebra[10]	1872
Prurigo gestationis	Besnier *et al.*[11]	1904
Erythema multiforme	Gross[12]	1930
Prurigo annularis	Davis[13]	1941
Toxemic rash of pregnancy	Bourne[14]	1962
Papular dermatitis of pregnancy	Spangler *et al*[15]	
Early and late-onset prurigo of pregnancy	Nurse[16]	1968
Pruritic urticarial papules and plaques of pregnancy	Lawley *et al.*[17]	1979
Pruritic folliculitis of pregnancy	Zoberman and Farmer[18]	1981

Table 4.3 The Specific Dermatoses of Pregnancy.

DERMATOSES OF PREGNANCY				
Diagnosis	**Clinical Signs**	**Laboratory Findings**	**Risks/ Complications**	**Management**
Pemphigoid (herpes) gestationis (See also Chapter 5)	erythema, wheals and blisters on abdomen (especially periumbilical), palms, soles, elsewhere	Immunofluoresence ++ (BMZ of skin and amnion)	mother: discomfort and increased risk of other auto-immune diseases fetus: blisters, increased risk of prematurity	prednisone, plasmaphoresis
Polymorphic eruption of pregnancy (See also Chapter 6)	papules, urticarial lesions on abdomen (common on striae distensae), thighs, buttocks, small vesicles may be present	Immunofluoresence -	none, other than mother's discomfort	topical corticosteroids
Prurigo of pregnancy (See also Chapter 7)	discrete erythematous papules on extremities, trunk	Immunofluoresence -	none, other than mother's discomfort	topical corticosteroids
Pruritic folliculitis of pregnancy (See also Chapter 7)	small, red follicular papules and pustules on back, arms ("acne")	Immunofluoresence -	mother: discomfort fetus: none	5% benzoyl peroxide +, 1% hydrocortisone
COMMON SKIN DISORDERS WHICH MAY MIMIC DERMATOSES OF PREGNANCY				
Allergic				
Urticaria (Hives) Drug reactions Contact dermatitis	Does not blister, lesions transient Ingestion of medication Pattern, history of allergen			
Common Skin Eruptions				
Atopic dermatitis/eczema	Family history of asthma, hay fever, rash on antecubital/popliteal folds, comes and goes with seasons, very itchy and chronic			
Pityriasis rosea	Oval, slightly scaly plaques on trunk, "herald patch" may precede rash by 1–2 weeks. May mimic secondary syphilis, consider serum test for syphilis			
Erythema nodosum	Tender, red nodules on shins and lower legs, occasionally seen with pregnancy			
Miliaria	"Prickly heat", tiny vesicles on extremities/trunk in hot weather			
Insect bites and scabies	Flea bites are on legs most often, sometimes blister in sensitive patient. Scabies has linear papules in fingerwebs, elbows, aureolae			

Table 4.4 Differential Diagnoses of Dermatoses of Pregnancy.

3192 pregnant women with pruritus found that only seven cases could not be classified into a particular subgroup, according to the classification[22].

From time to time, 'new' disease entities are reported in the literature, but to date they remain essentially anecdotal single case reports. Impetigo herpetiformis, for example, is now considered to be a variant of pustular psoriasis (*see also Chapter 8*). Alcalay *et al.*[23] proposed the term linear IgM dermatosis of pregnancy, and described a single case of an intensely pruritic follicular papular eruption, which occurred in the third trimester. Linear deposition of IgM was noted at the dermoepidermal junction, but this disappeared after delivery. However, on clinical grounds, their case would have fitted well into the category of pruritic folliculitis of pregnancy.

CONCLUSION

It is clear that there is still much to be done in elucidating the pathogenesis of the specific dermatoses of pregnancy. Until this happens, the author suggests that the above proposed simplified clinical classification should be used. Such a method will usually provide sufficient clinical diagnostic information to advise and manage the patient. The following chapters deal with each of the specific dermatoses of pregnancy in greater detail.

REFERENCES

1 Fagan, E.A. Intrahepatic cholestasis of pregnancy. *B.M.J.* 1994; **309**:1242–1244.
2 Berg, B., Helm, G., Petersohn, L., *et al.* Cholestasis of pregnancy, clinical and laboratory studies. *Acta. Obstet. Gynecol. Scand.* 1986; **65**: 107–113.
3 Reyes, H. The spectrum of liver and gastrointestinal disease seen in cholestasis of pregnancy. *Gastroenterol. Clin. N. Am.* 1992; **21**: 905–921.
4 Shaw, D., Frohlich, J., Wittmann, B. A. K., *et al.* A prospective study of 18 patients with cholestasis of pregnancy. *Am. J. Obstet. Gynecol.* 1982; **142**: 621–625.
5 Rustgi, V. K. Liver disease in pregnancy. *Med. Clin. N. Am.* 1989; **73**: 1041–1047.
6 Reyes-Romero, M. A. Are changes in expression of actin genes involved in estrogen-induced cholestasis. *Med. Hypoth.* 1990; **32**: 39–43.
7 Fisk, N. M. and Bruce Storey, G. N. Fetal outcome in obstetric cholestasis. *Br. J. Obstet. Gynaecol.* 1988; **95**: 1137–1143.
8 Fisk, N. M., Bye, W. B., and Bruce Storey G. N. Maternal features of obstetric cholestasis: 20 years experience at King George V Hospital. *Aust. NZ. J. Obstet. Gynaecol.* 1988; **28**: 172–176.
9 Milton, J. L. *The Pathology and Treatment of Disease of the Skin.* Robert Hardwicke, London, 1872, p.205.
10 Hebra, F. Herpes impetiginiformis. *Lancet* 1872; **i**: 399–400.
11 Besnier, E., Brocq, L., and Jacquet, L. *la Pratique Dermatologique.* Masson et Cies, Paris, 1904, Vol. 1, p.75
12 Gross, P. Erythema multiforme gestationis. *Arch. Dermatol. Syph.* 1931; **23**: 567.
13 Davis, J. H. T. Prurigo annularis. *Br. J. Dermatol.* 1941; **53**: 143–145.
14 Bourne, G. Toxaemic rash of pregnancy. *Proc. R. Soc. Med.* 1962; **55**: 462–464.
15 Spangler, A. S., Reddy, W., Bardavil, W. A., *et al.* Papular dermatitis of pregnancy. *J.A.M.A.* 1962; **181**: 577–581.
16 Nurse, D. S. Prurigo of pregnancy. *Australas. J. Dermatol.* 1968; **9**: 258–267.
17 Lawley, T. J., Hertz, K. C., Wade, T. R., *et al.* Pruritic urticarial papules and plaques of pregnancy. *J.A.M.A.* 1979; **241**: 1696–1699.
18 Zoberman, E. and Farmer, E. R. Pruritic folliculitis of pregnancy. *Arch. Dermatol.* 1981; **117**: 20–22.
19 Holmes, R. C. and Black, M. M. The specific dermatoses of pregnancy: a reappraisal with special emphasis on a proposed simplied clinical classification. *Clin. Exp. Dermatol.* 1982; **7**: 65–73.
20 Holmes, R. C. and Black, M. M. The specific dermatoses of pregnancy. *J. Am. Acad. Dermatol.* 1983; **7**: 104–110.
21 Borradoni, L. and Saurat, J. H. Specific dermatoses of pregnancy: towards a comprehensive view? *Arch. Dermatol.* 1994; **130**: 778–780.
22 Roger, D., Vaillant, L., Fignon, A., *et al.* Specific pruritic diseases of pregnancy: a prospective study of 3,192 pregnant women. *Arch. Dermatol.* 1994; **130**: 734–739.
23 Alcalay, J., Ingber, A., Hazaz, B., *et al.* Linear IgM dermatosis of pregnancy. *J. Am. Acad. Dermatol.* 1988; **18**: 412–415.

5.
Pemphigoid (Herpes) Gestationis

Jeff K. Shornick

INTRODUCTION AND DEFINITION

Pemphigoid gestationis (PG) classically presents as a dramatic, vesiculobullous disease during pregnancy, usually in the second or third trimester, or in the immediate postpartum period. It has a typically characteristic onset, in which intensely pruritic, urticarial lesions on the abdomen progress rapidly to a generalized, pemphigoid-like, bullous eruption. The disorder may spontaneously improve during late pregnancy, but even if it does improve, it usually flares at the time of delivery. The disease usually regresses spontaneously in the weeks to months following delivery, but in a few cases, the disease may remain active for many years afterwards. The diversity of clinical features and the severity of clinical disease in PG have only recently become apparent.

Immunopathologically, PG is defined by the immunofluorescence (IF) demonstration of linear C3, with or without IgG, along the cutaneous basement membrane zone (BMZ). In most patients, indirect IF typically shows that the patient's serum can fix fresh C3 to cutaneous BMZ.

HISTORICAL BACKGROUND

The term herpes was first used by Galen (200 AD) in his description of the 'creeping eruptions' of cold sores associated with fever, and the spectrum of spreading, crusted eruptions. Milton (1872) coined the term herpes gestationis, applying it to a 'creeping eruption' associated with pregnancy. In retrospect, it is obvious that the condition had been reported earlier under other names. But in 1874 the term herpes gestationis was canonized by Buckley 'as embodying the clinical characters of the eruption and signifying at the same time the sex and state of the body in which it appears'.

However, considerable confusion was generated by the clinical and IF similarities between PG and bullous pemphigoid, and by the term herpes gestationis itself – particularly outside dermatology. In 1982, Holmes and Black therefore proposed that the disorder's name should be changed to pemphigoid gestationis[1]. Although this is now the preferred term in the UK and Europe, it is used very little in the USA, where the disorder is still usually called herpes gestationis (HG).

EPIDEMIOLOGY

Pemphigoid gestationis is undoubtedly a rare disease. Holmes et al.[2] found two cases among 84,000 deliveries in England, and Shornick et al.[3] estimated the incidence as 1 in 50,000 deliveries in the greater Dallas area. Even these incidences are probably overstated. The disease respects no racial boundaries, although evidence suggests that the incidence may vary according to the incidence of human leukocyte antigen (HLA)-DR4 in different population groups[4].

CLINICAL FEATURES

Pemphigoid gestationis may present during any pregnancy, not just the first one. It has also been reported with hydatidiform moles[5] and choriocarcinomas[6]. Once PG has developed in a pregnancy, it is generally thought to occur earlier and to be more severe during any subsequent pregnancy. However, in our studies of over 100 women with a history of PG, the clinical severity of PG does not seem to be predictable from the patient's previous history. Indeed, there have been recent reports of well-documented, disease-free pregnancies in women with a previous history of PG. Such 'skip pregnancies' comprise 5% of cases, and cannot be predicted by any clinical, epidemiologic, or laboratory features. Although certainly PG will recur in the great majority of cases, recurrence is not universal[3,7].

The disease typically presents with severe pruritus, which is soon followed by urticarial lesions during the second or third trimester. There have been reports of onset during the first trimester[8], but this is exceptional, even with recurrent disease. In 50% of cases, lesions begin on the abdomen, often within or immediately adjacent to the umbilicus (**5.1–5.3**). In the remaining 50% of patients, clinically typical lesions first erupt in an atypical distribution (e.g. the extremities, palms, or soles) (**5.4**). Progression to clustered, tense, vesiculobullous lesions on erythematous skin usually occurs within days to weeks of the initial onset of pruritus (**5.5–5.8**).

The classic description of PG is based upon the collective experience of the classic, mainly pre-IF, literature. Since the advent of IF techniques, it has become possible to approach PG from a different perspective. These techniques have shown that PG has an extremely variable clinical presentation and course. Clinically manifest PG occurs along a spectrum of disease from pruritic, urticarial disease without blisters at one end, to nearly universal, vesiculobullous involvement at

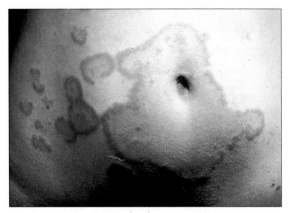

5.1 Early PG at 28 weeks' gestation. Pruritic polycyclic urticarial lesions have developed periumbilically.

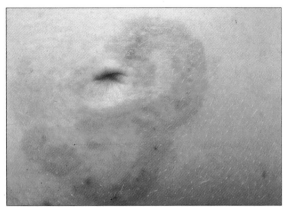

5.2 Early PG around the umbilicus. The urticarial lesions are beginning to develop vesicles.

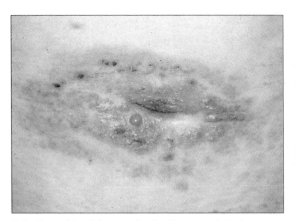

5.3 Pemphigoid gestationis. The periumbilical involvement is now clearly bullous.

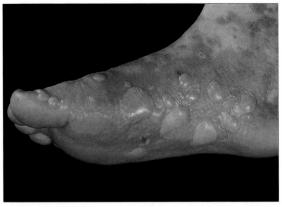

5.4 Pemphigoid gestationis. Large bullae developing on soles.

the other. PG may spontaneously resolve during the later part of gestation, only to flare at the time of delivery – such flaring occurs in at least 75% of patients.

About 25% of patients initially present within hours of parturition, after an otherwise uneventful pregnancy. The initial postpartum onset may be 'explosive', even within hours of delivery, but PG is an unlikely diagnosis if onset occurs more than three days postpartum. Other women may experience trivial, nonvesicular disease during one pregnancy, only to suffer exaggerated and characteristic bullous disease of PG during subsequent pregnancies.

As the disease begins to resolve, recurrences associated with the menstrual cycle are common. Recurrence may also develop during use of an oral contraceptive, and is seen in at least 25% of patients. There have been occasional reports of prolonged disease following delivery – which has even lasted years following parturition – but most patients experience spontaneous regression in the weeks to months following delivery, with or without treatment.

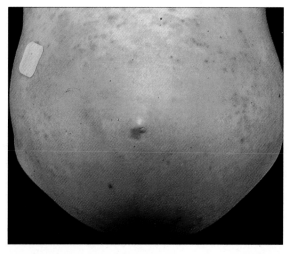

5.5 PG at 34 weeks' gestation. Pruritic urticarial lesions involve the entire abdomen.

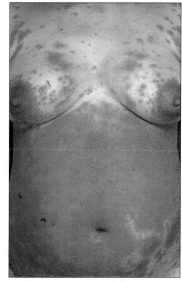

5.6 Pemphigoid gestationis. Pruritic urticarial lesions are spreading to involve the breasts.

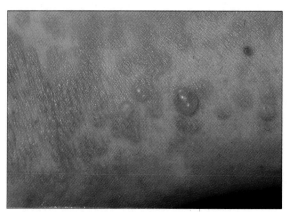

5.7 Pemphigoid gestationis. The same patient shown in **5.6**. Small bullae are developing within the areas of urticated erythema.

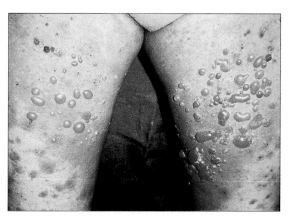

5.8 Severe PG, involving the anterior thighs.

DIFFERENTIAL DIAGNOSIS

The urticarial phase of PG may be confused with polymorphic eruption of pregnancy (PEP), a condition also known as pruritic urticarial papules and plaques of pregnancy (PUPPP). However, the rapid and relentless progression to vesiculobullous lesions generally makes PG an obvious diagnosis. The most common error in initial clinical assessment is to confuse PG with allergic contact dermatitis or drug eruptions. Immunofluorescence is the key to differential diagnosis, though the clinical course is usually sufficiently distinct to differentiate one disease from another.

INVESTIGATIONS

LABORATORY TESTS

Routine laboratory investigations tend to be uninformative. The correlation of peripheral eosinophilia with the severity of disease has been advocated[9], but has been difficult to confirm. Antinuclear antigens and complement levels are normal, while acute phase reactants may be increased. Most patients have circulating antiBMZ antibodies detectable by indirect complement-added IF, but the titer of circulating antiBMZ antibodies tends to be very low and does not correlate with either the extent or severity of disease. There is no apparent correlation between HLA type and the degree of clinical activity[10]. Although there is a nearly universal presence of antiHLA antibodies in patients with PG, there is no evidence that they are clinically relevant[11]. There is an increased incidence of antithyroid antibodies in patients with a history of PG[12], but clinically apparent thyroid dysfunction has rarely been reported concurrently with PG. Nevertheless, those with a history of PG are at increased risk of developing Graves' disease[12] (**5.9, 5.10**).

HISTOPATHOLOGY

The histopathology in PG classically shows a subepidermal vesicle, with lymphocytes and eosinophils in a perivascular distribution within the dermis (**5.11, 5.12**). Eosinophils may line up along the dermo–epidermal junction, and typically fill the vesicular space (eosinophilic spongiosis). However, a classical histopathology is rare, and changes are more likely to be non-specific, showing a mixed infiltrate, including eosinophils. Basal cell necrosis may be a prominent feature.

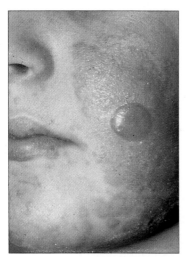

5.9 Severe PG, showing bulla and urticarial facial lesions.

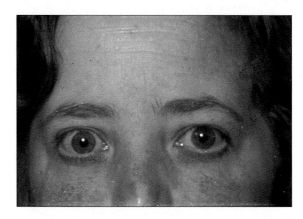

5.10 Thyrotoxicosis (Graves' disease) in the same patient shown in **5.9**. Thyrotoxicosis developed 10 years after the onset of severe PG.

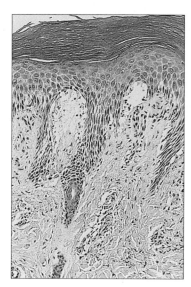

5.11 Histopathology of PG. Severe papillary dermal edema is present leading to early subepidermal separation. Eosinophils are present in the inflammatory infiltrate. (Hematoxylin & eosin stain x 4.)

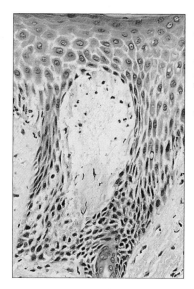

5.12 Histopathology of PG. Enlargement of section of **5.11**, showing an early vesicle. (Hematoxylin & eosin stain x 10.)

IMMUNOFLUORESCENCE FINDINGS

The *sine qua non* for the diagnosis of PG is the finding of linear C3 deposition during active disease, with or without IgG, along the BMZ of perilesional skin (**5.13**). The use of split-skin specimens, chemically separated along the lamina lucida, reveals that the immunoreactants are on the epidermal side.

Immunoelectron microscopy localizes immunoreactants to the lamina lucida, adjacent to the basal cell plasma membrane. In PG, IgG is detected by routine direct IF approximately 25% of the time, although it may be demonstrable more often if more refined multistep techniques are used[13,14]. Using indirect, complement-added IF, PG IgG can be detected in most cases. The PG IgG is directed towards a component of the hemidesmosomes, and shows preferential binding to a 180kDa protein over the 230–240kDa protein typically found in bullous pemphigoid (BP)[15,16]. However, some sera bind both antigens in both PG and BP. Recent evidence has shown that the 180kDa 'PG antigen' and the 240kDa 'BP antigen' are coded for by separate cDNAs[17] derived from separate chromosomes. Other evidence, produced by immunoelectron microscopy using immunogold techniques, suggests that the 180kDa PG antigen is a transmembrane protein, while the BP antigen is intracellular[18].

Pathophysiologically, the antibody fixes to the BMZ, triggering complement activation via the classical complement pathway. This results in chemoattraction of eosinophils and their subsequent degranulation. The release of proteolytic enzymes from eosinophilic granules is probably responsible for the resultant separation between epidermis and dermis.

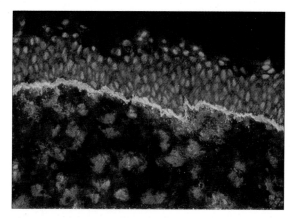

5.13 Direct immunofluorescence in PG. Bright linear deposition of C3 in the basement membrane zone.

IMMUNOGENETICS

As PG is exclusively a disease of pregnancy (or trophoblastic tumors), recent attention has focused on its immunogenetic basis, and the potential cross-reactivity between placental tissues and skin. Immunogenetic studies have revealed a marked increase in the HLA antigens DR3 and DR4:
- 61–80% of patients express DR3;
- 52–53% express DR4;
- 43–50% express both[10].

It is not known how these antigens contribute to the development of PG. However, as some patients do not express either antigen, although they have disease clinically indistinguishable from PG, the presence of characteristic HLA antigens alone is not sufficient to produce PG[10]. A mild increase in the HLA-DR2 antigen in the husbands of women with PG has been reported[19]. AntiHLA antibodies occur in essentially all those with a history of PG, compared to 25% of normal, multiparous controls[19], though the reasons for this are unclear.

PLACENTAL FINDINGS

It has recently been shown that the PG antibody binds to amniotic basement membrane[20,21] (**5.14**). This finding is not unexpected, since amnion is derived from fetal ectoderm and is antigenically similar to skin, with both pemphigoid and pemphigus antigens represented[22]. But there is a unique additional finding in the placental tissue of patients with PG.

Within the villous stroma of chorionic villi, adjacent to the maternal decidua, affected women show an increase in major histocompatibility complex (MHC) class II antigens (-DR, -DP, -DQ), together with an increased number of lymphocytes, near the site of immune attack[23–26]. This is not so in skin, where only complement components (with or without IgG) are seen along the BMZ[18,25]. Class II MHC antigens are not increased in skin.

These findings imply that the ongoing primary immune response may take place within the placenta. It has therefore been proposed that PG is a disease initiated by the aberrant expression of MHC class II antigens (of paternal haplotype). This causes an allogenic response to placental (amnion) BMZ, which cross-reacts with skin[27]. Much more research is needed to test this hypothesis, but based upon available data, such a proposition holds compelling interest.

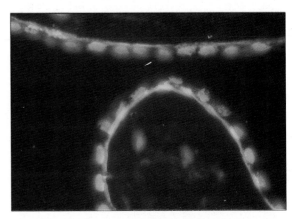

5.14 Placental immunology in PG. Linear binding of PG antibody to amniotic basement membrane.

HYDATIDIFORM MOLES AND CHORIOCARCINOMAS

Pemphigoid gestationis has been rarely reported in association with hydatidiform moles[5] and choriocarcinomas[6]. This is an intriguing clinical observation, because hydatidiform moles are most commonly produced by a diploid contribution of paternal chromosomes and have neither fetal tissue nor amnion.

There have also been no case reports of a PG-like dermatosis in males with choriocarcinoma. This malignancy is relatively common, and biochemically similar to normal pregnancy. Unlike choriocarcinomas in females, however, choriocarcinomas in males are entirely synergeneic. Placentae (and the moles derived from them) are primarily of paternal origin.

MATERNAL AND FETAL RISKS

The neonate may be affected with mild cutaneous involvement in up to 10% of cases, but the disease is typically self-limiting and resolves spontaneously over days to weeks. Transient urticarial or vesicular lesions are most common (**5.15**). Subclinical disease is probably common, as IF on fetal skin is routinely positive, despite a lack of clinically apparent disease.

There has been controversy about whether or not PG is associated with an increase in fetal morbidity or mortality. Kolodny[28] reviewed the pre-IF literature and concluded that there was 'no evidence supporting an increased incidence of stillbirth or abortion associated with PG'. However, Lawley *et al.*[9] reviewed 40 IF-confirmed PG cases taken primarily from the literature, and concluded that there was an increase in prematurity and stillbirth. However, this review has been criticized as relying too much upon reported cases. Another group of researchers, Shornick *et al.*[10] reported 28 previously unreported cases, identified by surveying the experience of IF laboratories, and were unable to confirm an increase in spontaneous abortions or stillbirths. Gestational age and birth weight, however, were not recorded.

Holmes *et al.*[29] studied an additional 33 cases and reported an increased incidence of small-for-gestational-age (SGA) births. The authors felt their findings suggested mild placental insufficiency in women with PG. A more recent study of 74 cases confirmed a slight tendency for SGA births and a tendency for prematurity in those pregnancies affected by PG[30]. The study found that 16% of deliveries occurred before 36 weeks, and that 32% of deliveries occurred before 38 weeks. However, in the same group of women, during pregnancies unaffected by PG, only 2% delivered before 36 weeks and 11% before 38 weeks[30]. The tendency for prematurity was not related to the use of systemic steroids, since there was no difference between those treated and those not treated.

No increases in spontaneous abortions or fetal mortality have been noted in any of the three studies published since Lawley's report[9]. Although the perception persists that there is significant fetal morbidity and mortality associated with PG, no such risk could be confirmed by any of the largest studies looking at this question.

ASSOCIATED DISEASES

Sporadic patients with PG have been reported to have additional autoimmune diseases (e.g. alopecia areata, Crohn's disease), but such reports are unusual. The exception is Graves' disease, which was present in 11% of 75 patients in the largest study on diseases associated with PG[12]. This study also documented a slight increase in other autoantibodies in patients with PG (or a history of PG), including antithyroid antibodies and gastric parietal cell antibodies. The study also found a 25% incidence of autoimmune diseases in the relatives of those with PG. Graves' disease was the most common autoimmune disease in relatives, but Hashimoto's thyroiditis and pernicious anemia were also noted. The secondary association of other autoimmune disease with PG is important and suggests that these patients should be assessed at regular intervals for the rest of their lives.

MANAGEMENT

The management of PG can be difficult, particularly while the patient is still pregnant. Topical corticosteroids are rarely useful once the vesiculobullous phase has developed. Systemic corticosteroids continue to be the mainstay of therapy and are generally safely prescribed in pregnancy. Prednisolone, 20–30mg daily, will control less severe cases, but at

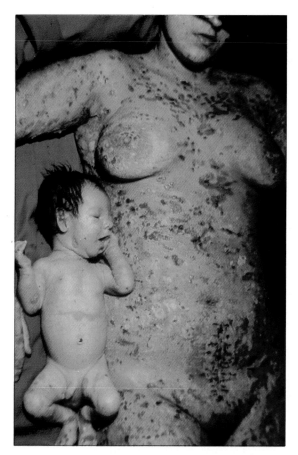

5.15 Mother to fetus transmission. The mother has severe PG, but only mild transient disease is present in the neonate.

times higher doses, 40–80mg daily, are needed to control severe disease. The dose of prednisolone can usually be tapered in the last trimester of pregnancy, but should be sharply increased soon after delivery to offset the almost inevitable postpartum flare of PG. After delivery, various adjuncts have been used, including dapsone, gold, and methotrexate, but none have proved beneficial. Plasmapheresis has been reported as beneficial in severe disease, but its use is clearly limited by logistics and expense[31].

Pemphigoid gestationis is clearly hormone-sensitive; 20–50% of women will experience an exacerbation with oral contraceptives. Exacerbations have been noted with both estrogens and progestogens, and many patients also experience regular pre-menstrual flares. A reversible chemical oophorectomy, using luteinizing hormone-releasing hormone analogues, has produced a remission in one woman with PG, who previously required large doses of prednisolone[32]. This therapeutic modality is worth exploring in chronic severe PG, but is clearly contraindicated in pregnancy.

REFERENCES

1 Holmes, R. C. and Black, M. M. The specific dermatoses of pregnancy: a reappraisal with special emphasis on a proposed simplified clinical classification. *Clin. Exp. Dermatol.* 1982; **7**: 65–73.
2 Holmes, R. C., Black, M. M., Dann, J., *et al.* A comparative study of toxic erythema of pregnancy, and herpes gestationis. *Br. J. Dermatol.* 1982; **106**: 499–510.
3 Shornick, J. K., Bangert, J. L., Freeman, R. G., *et al.* Herpes gestationis: clinical and histologic features of 28 cases. *J. Am. Acad. Dermatol.* 1983; **8**: 214–224.
4 Shornick, J. K., Meek, T. J., Nesbit, L. T., *et al.* Herpes gestationis in blacks. *Arch. Dermatol.* 1984: **120**: 511–513.
5 Tindall, J. G., Rea, T. H., Shulman, I., *et al.* Herpes gestationis in association with hydatidiform mole: immunopathologic studies. *Arch. Dermatol.* 1981; **117**: 510–512.
6 Siazinski, L. and Degefu, S. Herpes gestationis associated with choriocarcinoma. *Arch. Dermatol.* 1982; **118**: 425–428.
7 Holmes, R. C., Black, M. M., Jurecka, W., *et al.* Clues to the aetiology and pathogenesis of herpes gestationis. *Br. J. Dermatol.* 1983; **109**: 131–139.
8 Coupe, R. L. Herpes gestationis. *Arch. Dermatol.* 1965; **91**: 633–666.
9 Lawley, T. J., Stingl, G., and Katz, S. L. Fetal and maternal risk factors in herpes gestationis. *Arch. Dermatol.* 1978; **114**: 552–555.
10 Shornick, J. K., Stasny, P., and Gillam, J. N. High frequency of histocompatibility antigens HLA-DR3 and DR4 in herpes gestationis. *J. Clin. Invest.* 1981; **68**: 553–555.
11 Shornick, J. K., Jenkins, R. E., Briggs, D. C., *et al.* Anti-HLA antibodies in pemphigoid gestationis. *Br. J. Dermatol.* 1993; **129**: 257–259.
12 Shornick, J. K. and Black, M. M. Secondary autimmune diseases in herpes gestationis (pemphigoid gestationis). *J. Am. Acad. Dermatol.* 1992; **26**: 563–566.
13 Holubar, K., Konrad, K., and Stingl, G. Detection by immunoelectron microscopy of immunoglobulin G deposits in skin of immunofluorescent-negative herpes gestationis. *Br. J. Dermatol.* 1977; **96**: 569–571.
14 Karpati, S., Stolz, W., Meurer, M., *et al.* Herpes gestationis: ultrastructural identification of the extracellular antigenic sites in diseased skin using immunogold techniques. *Br. J. Dermatol.* 1991; **125**: 317–324.
15 Kelly, S. E., Bhogal, B. S., Wojnarowska, F., *et al.* Western blot analysis of the antigen in pemphigoid gestationis. *Br. J. Dermatol.* 1990; **122**: 445–449.
16 Morrison, L. H., Labib, R. S., Zone, J. J., *et al.* Herpes gestationis autoantibodies recognize a 180-kD human epidermal antigen. *J. Clin. Invest.* 1988; **81**: 2023–2026.
17 Diaz, L. A., Ratrie, H. III, Saunders, W. S., *et al.* Isolation of a human epidermal cDNA corresponding to the 180 kD autoantigen recognized by bullous pemphigoid and herpes gestationis sera. Immunolocalization of this protein to the hemidesmosome. *J. Clin. Invest.* 1990; **86**: 1088–1094.
18 Mutasim, D. F., Takahashi, Y., Labib, R. S., *et al.* A pool of bullous pemphigoid antigen(s) is intracellular and associated with the basal cell cytoskeleto-hemidesmosome complex. *J. Invest. Dermatol.* 1985; **84**: 47–53.
19 Shornick, J. K., Artlett, C. M., Jenkins, R. E., *et al.* Complement polymorphism in herpes gestationis (pemphigoid gestationis): association with C4 null allele. *J. Am. Acad. Dermatol.* 1993; **29**: 545–549.
20 Kelly, S. E., Bhogal, B. S., Wojnarowska, F., *et al.* Expression of pemphigoid gestationis-related antigen by human placenta. *Br. J. Dermatol.* 1988; **118**: 605–611.
21 Ortonne, J. P., Hsi, B. L., Verando, P., *et al.* Herpes gestationis factor reacts with the amniotic epithelial basement membrane. *Br. J. Dermatol.* 1987; **117**: 147–154.
22 Robinson, H. N., Anhalt, G., Patel, H. P., *et al.* Pemphigus and pemphigoid antigens are expressed in human amnion epithelium. *J. Invest. Dermatol.* 1984; **83**: 234–237.
23 Borthwick, G. M., Sunderland C. H., Holmes, R. C., *et al.* Abnormal expression of HLA-DR antigen in the placenta of a patient with pemphigoid gestationis. *J. Repro. Immunol.* 1984; **6**: 393–396.
24 Borthwick, G. M., Holmes, R. C., and Stirrat, G. M. Abnormal expression of class II MHC antigens in placentae from patients with pemphigoid gestationis: analysis of class II MHC subregion product expression. *Placenta* 1988; **9**: 81–94.
25 Kelly, S. E., Fleming, S., Bhogal, B. S., *et al.* Immunopathology of the placenta in pemphigoid gestationis and linear IgA disease. *Br. J. Dermatol.* 1989; **120**: 735–743.
26 Kelly, S. E., Black, M. M., and Fleming, S. Antigen-presenting cells in the skin and placenta in pemphigoid gestationis. *Br. J. Dermatol.* 1990; **122**: 593–599.
27 Kelly, S. E., Black, M. M., and Fleming, S. Pemphigoid gestationis: a unique mechanism of initiation of an autoimmune response by MHC class II molecules? *J. Pathol.* 1989; **158**: 81–82.
28 Kolodny, R. C. Herpes gestationis: a new assessment of incidence, diagnosis, and fetal prognosis. *Am. J. Obstet. Gynecol.* 1969: **104**: 39–45.
29 Holmes R. C. and Black, M. M. The fetal prognosis in pemphigoid gestationis (herpes gestationis). *Br. J. Dermatol.* 1984; **110**: 67–72.
30 Shornick, J. K. and Black, M. M. Fetal risks in herpes gestationis. *J. Am. Acad. Dermatol.* 1992; **26**: 63–68.
31 Van de Weil, A., Hart, H. C., Flinterman, J., *et al.* Plasma exchange in herpes gestationis. *Br. Med. J.* 1908; **281**: 1041–1042.
32 Garvey, M. P., Handfield-Jones, S. E., and Black, M. M. Pemphigoid gestationis – response to chemical oophorectomy with goserelin. *Clin. Exp. Dermatol.* 1992; **17**: 443–445.

ACKNOWLEDGEMENT

Figure **5.15** has been reproduced by kind permission of Professor Ernesto Bonifazi, Bari, Italy.

6.
Polymorphic Eruption of Pregnancy

Martin M. Black

INTRODUCTION

Polymorphic eruption of pregnancy (PEP) is probably the most common of the gestational dermatoses, affecting about one in 160 pregnancies. It is essentially a self-limiting, papular, urticarial eruption of late pregnancy and/or the puerperium. A few cases may develop vesicles or smaller bullae, target lesions, polycyclic wheals, and a widespread toxic erythema-like appearance.

HISTORICAL BACKGROUND

As PEP has a very variable clinical morphology[1], it is not surprising that various terms have been used to describe it. The disease was initially reported as 'toxemic rash of pregnancy'[2], but as the case was not associated with pre-eclampsia the term was little used. Since then other descriptive terms have been used, including prurigo of late pregnancy[3], toxic erythema of pregnancy[4], and pruritic urticarial papules and plaques of pregnancy (PUPPP)[5,6].

Although the term PUPPP is still widely used, particularly in the USA, it is generally agreed that PUPPP and PEP are identical dermatoses[7]. We prefer to use PEP, because it encapsulates the full range of clinical morphologic expressions, including papules, plaques, target lesions, polycyclic erythematous wheals, vesicles, and occasional bullae.

ETIOLOGY

Polymorphic eruption of pregnancy is an inflammatory dermatosis associated solely with pregnancy. No associations have been found with atopy, pre-eclampsia, or autoimmune phenomena[1], and the frequency of human lymphocyte antigens (HLA) in women with PEP is also normal[1,6]. The common clinical presentation of PEP in abdominal striae suggests that abdominal distension may be an important factor. A reaction to abdominal distension has also been implicated by the greater likelihood in PEP of higher maternal weight gain, higher neonatal birth weight, and increased incidence of twins[8,9].

No evidence has been found to implicate autoimmune or hormonal mechanisms in PEP[10,11]. Circulating immune complexes have also not been found in PEP[6]. Although PEP is now a well-recognized entity, it is perhaps surprising that there is little substantial information about its etiology, and factors such as parity, multiple pregnancy and paternity may well need further consideration[12].

CLINICAL FEATURES

The great majority of cases with PEP are primigravidas, and the development of PEP in a subsequent pregnancy is very likely to coexist with excessive maternal weight gain or multiple pregnancies[13]. The characteristic time of onset is between the 36th and 39th week of gestation, but lesions can also develop in the immediate postpartum period. There is no particular maternal age at which PEP is likely to develop[6].

The mean duration of the eruption is six weeks, but the eruption is usually not severe for more than one week[1]. The eruption begins with pruritic urticarial papules, usually in association with striae distensae (**6.1–6.3**); however, these papules can develop on the abdomen without striae (**6.4**). Earlier reports of PEP indicated that the lesions consisted almost exclusively of urticarial papules and plaques[5]. However, the morphology of the eruption may vary greatly throughout its duration[1]. Forty per cent of cases develop tiny vesicles, often on top of the papules overlying striae (**6.5**). Target-like lesions are present in 20% of cases (**6.6**) and annular or polycyclic wheals in 18% (**6.6**). In 70% of cases, the lesions become confluent and widespread, resembling a toxic erythema (**6.7**). In a small number of cases, vesicles may coalesce to form smaller bullae[14] (**6.8**). The Koebner or isomorphic response in PEP is common[15],

but facial involvement is very rare[15,16]. As the eruption slowly resolves, the great majority of cases exhibit fine scaling and crusting, suggestive of eczema[1].

The eruption begins on the lower abdomen, but often spares the periumbilical area (**6.1**, **6.2**). Other commonly affected sites include the thighs, buttocks (**6.9**), and the extensor surfaces of the arms (**6.10**). It is most unusual to see the hands and feet affected, but if they are, the condition may resemble scabies (**6.11**) Mucosal lesions have not been described. In more severe PEP, the erythema may confluently involve the entire abdomen, thighs, and even elsewhere (**6.12**).

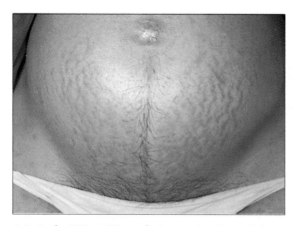

6.1 Early PEP at 38 weeks' gestation in an Asian primigravida. Pruritic urticaria in striae distensae. Note the periumbilical sparing.

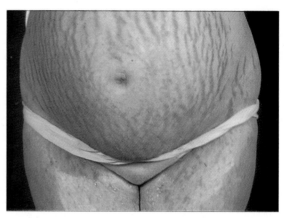

6.2 PEP at 37 weeks in a primigravida. Prominent pruritic urticarial lesions are present in striae distensae on abdomen and thighs.

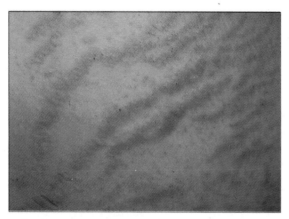

6.3 PEP in striae distensae. Close-up of **6.2**, showing confluent urticarial papules in striae distensae. Some papules occur adjacent to the striae.

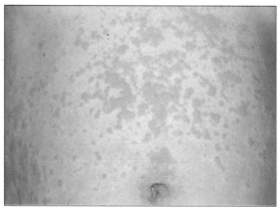

6.4 PEP at 36 weeks' gestation in a primigravida. Urticarial papules on the upper abdomen in the absence of striae distensae.

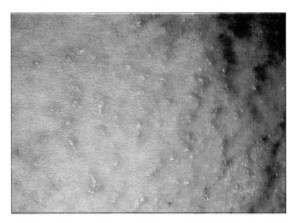

6.5 PEP morphology. 'Pinpoint-sized' vesicles are present, on top of the urticarial papules within striae distensae.

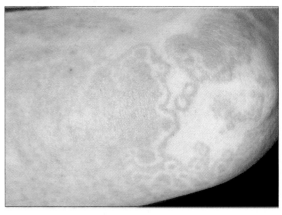

6.6 PEP morphology. 'Target-like' and annular polycyclic urticarial lesions around the elbow.

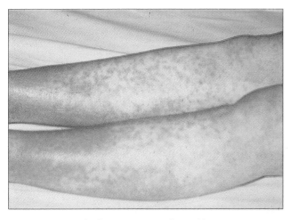

6.7 PEP morphology. Toxic erythema-like eruption on lower legs.

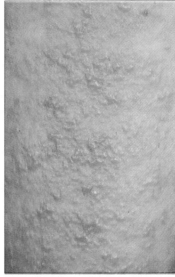

6.8 PEP morphology. Vesiculobullous eruption on lower legs.

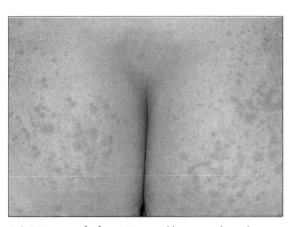

6.9 PEP morphology. Urticarial lesions on buttocks.

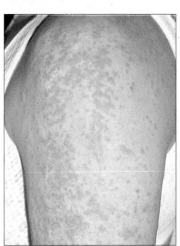

6.10 PEP morphology. Urticarial lesions on upper arms.

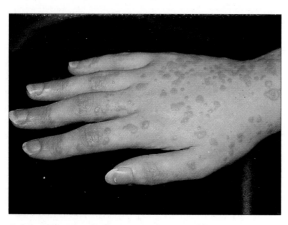

6.11 PEP morphology. Acral urticarial lesions resembling scabies.

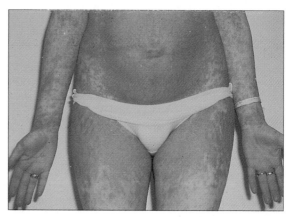

6.12 Severe PEP. In this patient, the abdomen, thighs, and forearms are involved.

HISTOPATHOLOGY AND IMMUNOFLUORESCENCE

Skin biopsies for routine histopathology usually reveal a superficial and mid-dermal, perivascular, lymphohistiocytic infiltrate, with a variable number of eosinophils present. Spongiosis, parakeratosis and marked papillary dermal edema may be present leading to subepidermal vesicle formation[17] (**6.13**). These histopathologic changes in PEP may overlap with those seen in pemphigoid gestationis (PG).

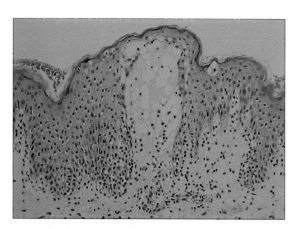

6.13 Histology of PEP. Focal spongiosis is evident with a small subepidermal vesicle. The inflammatory infiltrate contains a few eosinophils. (Hematoxylin & eosin stain x10.)

Direct immunofluorescence (DIF) is negative in the great majority of PEP cases. However, some investigators have reported equivocal DIF findings in PEP, such as minimal C3 deposition along the basement membrane zone, perivascular C3 and fibrin in the dermis[6,18], and in one case antiepidermal cell surface antibodies[19]. Saurat[20] has stressed the importance of performing DIF in PEP, because some cases of PEP may be very similar clinically to PG.

DIFFERENTIAL DIAGNOSIS

Since PEP may have a variable clinical morphology, it may be confused with several disorders, including drug eruptions, pemphigoid gestationis, scabies, and erythema multiforme. The following comparison may help to differentiate between PEP and PG:

- Examination of striae distensae is important since lesions overlying striae are found in 90% of PEP cases[1], but are seldom prominent in PG.
- Although vesicles are found in 40% of PEP cases, they are unlikely to be larger than 2–3 mm in diameter. However, once vesicles occur in PG, they usually rapidly evolve into larger tense bullae.
- Involvement of periumbilical skin is a common finding (84%) in PG, but is only observed in 10% of PEP cases[1].

Nevertheless, we firmly recommend that DIF is performed on all cases of PEP to avoid any diagnostic confusion with PG.

PROGNOSIS

Apart from the discomfort of the pruritic urticarial eruption, the maternal prognosis is unaffected. However, the number of twin pregnancies in PEP appears to be significantly increased[8]. Carruther's experience indicated that resolution of the eruption in PEP appeared to be unrelated to delivery of the infant[21], and it is generally agreed that fetal prognosis is normal[1,5,6,10,18]. Only one possible case of transient neonatal PEP involvement has been described[22].

MANAGEMENT

The disease is a self-limiting disorder without serious sequelae, and so only symptomatic treatment is usually required (**Table 6.1**). Most patients can obtain relief with the use of moderately potent topical corticosteroid creams (e.g. clobetasone butyrate, 0.05%, or hydrocortisone-17-butyrate, 0.01%), either singly or combined with small doses (4mg at night) of chlorpheniramine maleate. However, the new non-sedating antihistamines are not recommended in pregnancy[23]. More severe cases of PEP with a distressing degree of pruritus can be safely treated with oral prednisolone[9]. A tapering dose of prednisolone, 30mg daily for 7–14 days, should be sufficient. A severe case of PEP, unresponsive to therapy, was dramatically improved within two hours after cesarian section delivery[24].

Polymorphic eruption is the commonest gestational dermatosis, with an incidence of about one in 160 pregnancies

Onset is usually in the third trimester and in a primigravida

Lesions are commonly confined to striae distensae

Clinical morphology can be variable with urticarial papules, target-like lesions, polycyclic wheals and vesicles often seen

Direct immunofluorescence is negative

Eruption is self-limiting, seldom severe, and lasts about 1–4 weeks

Table 6.1 Polymorphic Eruption of Pregnancy – Key Points.

REFERENCES

1 Charles-Holmes, R. Polymorphic eruption of pregnancy. *Semin. Dermatol.* 1989; **8**: 18–22.

2 Bourne, G. Toxemic rash of pregnancy. *Proc. R. Soc. Med.* 1962; **55**: 462–464.

3 Nurse, D. S. Prurigo of pregnancy. *Aust. J. Dermatol.* 1968; **9**: 258–267.

4 Holmes, R. C., Black, M. M., Dann, J., *et al.* A comparative study of toxic erythema of pregnancy and herpes gestationis. *Br. J. Dermatol.* 1982; **106**: 499–510.

5 Lawley, T. J., Hertz, K. C., Wade, T. R., *et al.* Pruritic urticarial papules and plaques of pregnancy. *J. Am. Med. Assoc.* 1979; **241**: 1696–1699.

6 Yancey, K. B., Hall, R. P., and Lawley, T. J. Pruritic urticarial papules and plaques of pregnancy. *J. Am. Acad. Dermatol.* 1984; **10**: 473–480.

7 Alcalay, J. and Wolf, J. E. Pruritic urticarial papules and plaques of pregnancy: the enigma and the confusion. *J. Am. Acad. Dermatol.* 1988; **19**: 1115–1116.

8 Cohen, L. M., Capeless, E. L., Krusinski, P. A., *et al.* Pruritic urticarial papules and plaques of pregnancy and its relationship to maternal–fetal weight gain and twin pregnancy. *Arch. Dermatol.* 1989; **125**: 1534–1536.

9 Bunker, C. B., Erskine, K., Rustin, M. H. A., *et al.* Severe polymorphic eruption of pregnancy occurring in twin pregnancies. *Clin. Exp. Dermatol.* 1990; **15**: 228–231.

10 Alcalay, J., Ingber, A., Kafri, B., *et al.* Hormonal evaluation and autoimmune background in pruritic urticarial papules and plaques of pregnancy. *Am. J. Obstet. Gynecol.* 1988; **158**: 417–420.

11 Callen, J. P. and Hanno, R. Pruritic urticarial papules and plaques of pregnancy (PUPPP): a clinicopathologic study. *J. Am. Acad. Dermatol.* 1981; **5**: 401–405.

12 Powell, F. C. Parity, polypregnancy, paternity and PUPPP. *Arch. Dermatol.* 1992; **128**: 1551.

13 Beckett, M. A. and Goldberg, N. S. Pruritic urticarial plaques and papules of pregnancy and skin distension. *Arch. Dermatol.* 1991; **127**: 125–126.

14 Holmes, R. C., McGibbon, D. H., and Black, M. M. Polymorphic eruption of pregnancy with subepidermal vesicles. *J. R. Soc. Med.* 1984; **77**: 22–23.

15 Carruthers, A. Facial involvement in pruritic urticarial papules and plaques of pregnancy. *J. Am. Acad. Dermatol.* 1987; **17**: 302.

16 Alcalay, J., David, M., and Sandbank, M. Facial involvement in pruritic urticarial papules and plaques of pregnancy. *J. Am. Acad. Dermatol.* 1986; **15**: 1048.

17 Holmes, R. C., Jureka, W., and Black, M. M. A comparative histopathological study of polymorphic eruption of pregnancy and herpes gestationis. *Clin. Exp. Dermatol.* 1983; **8**: 523–529.

18 Alcalay, J., Ingber, A., David, M., *et al.* Pruritic urticarial papules and plaques of pregnancy: a review of 21 cases. *J. Reprod. Med.* 1987; **32**: 315–316.

19 Trattner, A., Ingber, A., and Sandbank, M. Antiepidermal cell surface antibodies in a patient with pruritic urticarial papules and plaques of pregnancy. *J. Am. Acad. Dermatol.* 1991; **24**: 306–308.

20 Saurat, J. H. Immunofluorescence biopsy for pruritic urticarial papules and plaques of pregnancy. *J. Am. Acad. Dermatol.* 1989; **20**: 711.

21 Carruthers, A. Pruritic urticarial papules and plaques of pregnancy. *J. Am. Acad. Dermatol.* 1993; **29**: 125.

22 Uhlin, S. R. Pruritic urticarial papules and plaques of pregnancy. Involvement of the mother and infant. *Arch. Dermatol.* 1981; **117**: 238–239.

23 Jurecka, W. and Gebhart, W. Drug prescribing during pregnancy. *Semin. Dermatol.* 1989; **8**: 30–39.

24 Beltrani, V. P. and Beltrani, V. S. Pruritic urticarial papules and plaques of pregnancy: a severe case requiring early delivery for relief of symptoms. *J. Am. Acad. Dermatol.* 1992; **26**: 266–267.

7.
Prurigo of Pregnancy, Papular Dermatitis of Pregnancy, and Pruritic Folliculitis of Pregnancy

Martin M. Black

INTRODUCTION

These three disease entities are described in the same chapter because each term applying is still widely used in the literature. There may be overlap between them and there is considerable doubt that they are all distinct clinical entities. All three conditions are characterized by discrete, pruritic papules, which soon become excoriated. This chapter will outline the clinical and differentiating features of each entity.

PRURIGO OF PREGNANCY

HISTORICAL BACKGROUND

In 1904, Besnier[1] first introduced the term 'prurigo gestationis' to include all patients with pregnancy-related dermatoses, other than those with herpes gestationis. Costello, in 1941[2], estimated that 'prurigo

gestationis of Besnier' occurred in 2% of pregnancies. In 1968, Nurse[3] outlined the clinical features of prurigo of pregnancy, but also included cases of polymorphic eruption of pregnancy under this term ('late-onset' prurigo of pregnancy).

CLINICAL FEATURES

Prurigo of pregnancy is not uncommon and affects about one in 300 pregnancies[3]. The onset is usually about 25–30 weeks' gestation, and it can persist for up to three months postpartum. The lesions are discrete erythematous or skin-colored papules, which are extremely pruritic, with the result that an excoriated surface soon develops over the papules. The papules tend to be small and are seldom larger than 0.5cm in diameter. Usually, the lesions remain papular, and thus the surrounding skin does not develop features of eczema. Characteristically, the papules appear on the extensor surfaces of the extremities and trunk, and do not progress to vesicle formation[4] (**7.1–7.3**). There is little follow-up

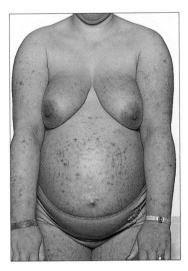

7.1 Prurigo of pregnancy. Diffuse prurigo papules scattered on the abdomen and extensor limb surfaces. The condition closely simulates 'papular dermatitis of pregnancy'.

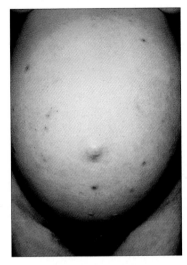

7.2 Prurigo of pregnancy. Discrete excoriated papules on the abdomen in late pregnancy.

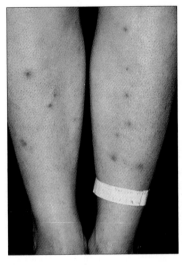

7.3 Prurigo of pregnancy. Same patient as in **7.2**, showing excoriated papules on the lower legs.

information on the reappearance of prurigo of pregnancy in subsequent pregnancies. Hayashi[4] believes it to be a rare occurrence.

The histologic features of prurigo of pregnancy have not been studied systematically, and consequently at present the diagnosis is made on clinical criteria alone. Where biopsies have been performed, the pathology usually shows mild acanthosis, parakeratosis, and surface excoriation. A mixed perivascular infiltrate is found, often containing eosinophils and some neutrophils[5]. Direct immunofluorescence (DIF) is negative[5].

PATHOGENESIS

Prurigo of pregnancy is perhaps the least studied of all the dermatoses of pregnancy. However, Holmes and Black[5] have postulated that prurigo of pregnancy might simply be the result of pruritus gravidarum occurring in atopic women. They base their argument on the finding that 18% of pregnancies are complicated by pruritus[6] and that 10% of the population display atopy[7]. It might therefore be expected that both conditions would coincide in about 2% of pregnancies.

TREATMENT

Prurigo of pregnancy is a benign disorder, but the patient may find the persistent pruritus distressing. Symptomatic relief of pruritus usually can be achieved using moderately potent topical corticosteroid creams, such as Class 4 or 5 clobetasone butyrate, 0.05% cream, or hydrocortisone-17-butyrate, 0.1% cream, with oral chlorpheniramine maleate, 4mg at night. The use of Cordran tape (translucent polythene adhesive film impregnated with flurandrenolone) can be effective in the management of a smaller number of discrete, pruritic papules.

PAPULAR DERMATITIS OF PREGNANCY

Papular dermatitis of pregnancy was first described by Spangler *et al.*[8] in 1962. They identified a group of patients, whom they thought could be differentiated from prurigo of pregnancy, both clinically and biochemically. They stressed the high fetal risk which they considered to be preventable by appropriate therapy. There is considerable doubt, however, that papular dermatitis of pregnancy is an entity separate from more widespread examples of prurigo of pregnancy. Nor is it likely that the disorder carries an appreciable fetal risk[9].

CLINICAL FEATURES

Spangler *et al.*[8] originally described 12 cases of papular dermatitis. The eruption occurred throughout pregnancy from 11 weeks' gestation to term. The condition was described as a generalized papular eruption over the trunk, arms, legs, and even the face. The papules were 3–5mm in diameter and excoriated. Rahbari[10] later described 16 cases and noted that the papules could have an erythematous, urticated appearance, prior to excoriation.

Spangler *et al.*[8] estimated an incidence of about one in 2400 pregnancies and expressed concern about the high level of fetal mortality (27–37%). In recent years, very few new cases of papular dermatitis have been reported[11,12]. The similarity of the eruption to prurigo of pregnancy[9] (**7.1**) and pruritic folliculitis of pregnancy has been noted[12].

HISTOPATHOLOGY

The histopathologic findings in papular dermatitis have mainly been studied by Rahbari[10]. They clearly overlap with those of prurigo of pregnancy[5], with the following features occurring in both.
• Epidermal acanthosis;
• Excoriation;
• A perivascular accumulation of eosinophils and neutrophils.
The few DIF observations made in papular dermatitis have been negative[12].

BIOCHEMISTRY

Spangler *et al.*[8,13] reported elevated chorionic gonadotrophin, lowered plasma cortisol levels, and reduced urinary estriol levels in papular dermatitis of pregnancy. These findings were also reported subsequently in individual case reports[11,12]. Unfortunately, to date, no systematic study has compared the above potential biochemical abnormalities of papular dermatitis with the more common and similar condition of prurigo of pregnancy.

TREATMENT

Due to the increased fetal mortality they found, Spangler *et al.*[8] recommended systemic administration of either prednisone (prednisolone), up to 200mg daily, or diethystilbestrol, 600–2500mg daily. They claimed that these therapies cleared the dermatosis within a few days and reversed the potential fetal loss. However, subsequently, Rahbari[10] did not find a high fetal loss and recommended 'conservative treatment'. Individual case reports have reported on the beneficial use of tapering doses of prednisone[11,12].

REAPPRAISAL

A comprehensive reappraisal of the startling claims of Spangler *et al.*[8,13] has cast considerable doubt on the nosology of papular dermatitis[5]. The author's view is that clinically their cases of papular dermatitis represent more widespread and severe cases of prurigo of pregnancy[9]. The main reason for the separate classification of papular dermatitis of pregnancy was based on the findings of raised urinary chorionic gonadotrophin, low urinary cortisol and low urinary estriol[8,13]. However, it is important to stress that similar biochemical studies were not performed in any other dermatoses of pregnancy. This important question about the validity of papular dermatitis of pregnancy cannot be resolved until biochemical data on the other pregnancy dermatoses become available.

Furthermore, the fetal mortality in the original report of Spangler *et al.*[8] was probably overestimated for the following reasons.

- The interpretation of fetal deaths that occurred in pregnancies preceding the development of papular dermatitis was not justified, and exaggerated the fetal risk.
- Their data included spontaneous abortions without reference to the period of gestation. This is important because first-trimester spontaneous abortions are not uncommon in a normal population.

There would therefore seem to be considerable doubt about whether papular dermatitis of pregnancy is an entity entirely separate from the more common condition of prurigo of pregnancy.

PRURITIC FOLLICULITIS OF PREGNANCY

The term 'pruritic folliculitis of pregnancy' was first introduced by Zoberman and Farmer in 1981[14]. They described six patients who had developed a pruritic, follicular papular eruption between the fourth and ninth months of pregnancy, which then resolved within 2–3 weeks of delivery. The lesions were principally small, follicular erythematous papules or pustules,

distributed widely over the upper trunk. Histopathologic findings were interpreted as an acute folliculitis, but unfortunately no biochemical findings were presented. However, the clinical descriptions of pruritic folliculitis of pregnancy suggest that the eruption can mimic papular dermatitis[12].

The author has seen a number of patients with a similar widespread eruption consisting of small erythematous papules and pustules (**7.4, 7.5**). Topical treatment with a cream containing benzoyl peroxide, 10%, and hydrocortisone, 1%, was beneficial. The author's view is that the clinical appearance of pruritic folliculitis of pregnancy is very similar to the monomorphic type of acne occurring after the administration of systemic corticosteroids or progestogens[5]. It is therefore possible that pruritic folliculitis of pregnancy is a form of hormonally induced acne rather than a specific dermatosis of pregnancy.

7.4 Pruritic folliculitis of pregnancy. Diffuse small monormorphic acneiform papules and pustules present on the patient's back.

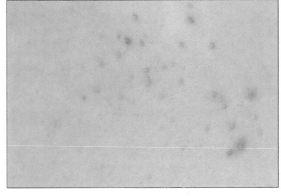

7.5 Pruritic folliculitis of pregnancy. A close-up of **7.4** shows small follicular papules and pustules.

REFERENCES

1 Besnier, E., Brocq, L., and Jacquet, L. *La Pratique Dermatologique.* Masson et Cie, Paris, 1975, Vol. 1, p.75.

2 Costello, M. J. Eruptions of pregnancy. *New York State J. Med.* 1941; **41**: 849–855.

3 Nurse, D. S. Prurigo of pregnancy. *Australas. J. Dermatol.* 1968; **9**: 258–267.

4 Hayashi, R. H. Bullous dermatoses and prurigo of pregnancy. *Clin. Obstet. Gynecol.* 1990; **33**: 746–753.

5 Holmes, R. C. and Black, M. M. The specific dermatoses of pregnancy. *J. Am. Acad. Dermatol.* 1983; **8**: 405–412.

6 Kasdon, S. C. Abdominal pruritus in pregnancy. *Am. J. Obstet. Gynecol.* 1953; **65**: 320–324.

7 Rapaport, H. G., Appel, S. J., and Szanton V.L. Incidence of allergy in a pediatric population. *Am. J. Allergy* 1960; **18**: 45–49.

8 Spangler, A. S., Reddy, W., Bardawill, W. A., *et al.* Papular dermatitis of pregnancy. *J. Am. Med. Assoc.* 1962; **181**: 577–581.

9 Black, M. M. Prurigo of pregnancy, papular dermatitis of pregnancy and pruritic folliculitis of pregnancy. *Semin. Dermatol.* 1989; **8**: 23–25.

10 Rahbari, H. Pruritic papules of pregnancy. *J. Cutan. Pathol.* 1978; **5**: 347–352.

11 Michaund, R. M., Jacobson, D., and Dahl, M. V. Papular dermatitis of pregnancy. *Arch. Dermatol.* 1982; **118**: 1003–1005.

12 Nguyen, L. Q. and Sarmini, O. R. Papular dermatitis of pregnancy: a case report. *J. Am. Acad. Dermatol.* 1990; **22**: 690–691.

13 Spangler, A. S. and Emerson, K. Estrogen levels and estrogen therapy in papular dermatitis of pregnancy. *Am. J. Obstet. Gynecol.* 1971; **110**: 534–537.

14 Zoberman, E. and Farmer, E. R. Pruritic folliculitis of pregnancy. *Arch. Dermatol.* 1981; **117**: 20–22.

8.
Effect of Pregnancy on Other Skin Disorders

Rachel E. Jenkins & Martin M. Black

INTRODUCTION

Pregnancy causes immunologic, endocrine, metabolic, and vascular changes in the pregnant woman which modify her responses to skin diseases. Both the obstetrician and the dermatologist need to be aware of this potential if they are to provide optimal management during pregnancy. Particular attention should be given to any medication administered to a pregnant or nursing woman; the reader is advised to consult published guidelines and/or review articles[1,2,3,4,5].

ECZEMA

Atopic eczema is a chronic, relapsing, pruritic dermatitis, affecting 1–5% of the general population. About 75–80% of patients with atopic eczema have a personal or family history of allergic disease. *Acute eczema* results in intensely pruritic, erythematous papules and vesicles, or extensive erosions with serous exudate. *Subacute eczema* is more organized and is most often associated with excoriated, scaling and erythematous papules or plaques, grouped or scattered over erythematous skin. *Chronic eczema* is characterized by thickened, lichenified skin (**8.1**).

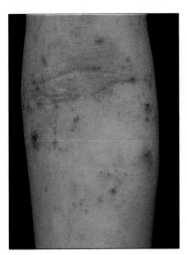

8.1 Eczema. Lichenified skin with excoriations in antecubital fossa in chronic atopic eczema.

MANAGEMENT

A patient with eczema should try to avoid local heat and contact with irritants such as soap and detergents. The mainstay of treatment is keeping the skin moisturized with frequent use of topical emollients and bath-oils. Topical emollients should also be applied during the day, between steroid applications. It is important to find an emollient that suits the individual patient. There are many available, ranging from white soft paraffin (Vaseline), which is very greasy, to aqueous cream which is not greasy. Patients should also soak for 10–15 minutes daily in a lukewarm bath, with bath-oil added as a moisturizer. Emulsifying ointment or aqueous cream should be used as a soap substitute.

PREGNANCY

The pregnant patient with atopic eczema should use only the weakest possible topical corticosteroid for routine maintenance, but in acute exacerbations, high potency Class 1 or 2 corticosteroids may be applied for a few days, with a slow return to a low potency steroid. Ointments rather than creams should be used to prevent loss of water from the skin. The adverse effects of topical corticosteroids include skin atrophy, depigmentation, acneiform papules and, rarely, systemic effects. Tar-containing preparations, such as crude coal tar, are useful in treating eczema and are safe to use in pregnancy.

Occasionally, systemic corticosteroids, such as prednisone (prednisolone), are required for a short period in acute eczema. Prednisone, 30mg daily, may be required initially, with the dose tapered over one week. Although fetal cleft palate has been reported, prednisone is probably safe to use in pregnancy. However, fetal or neonatal adrenal suppression may occur with continuous therapy greater than 10mg of prednisone daily. Small amounts of corticosteroids also pass into the breast milk, though low doses of prednisone, e.g. 5mg daily, are unlikely to have an adverse effect on the infant. The patient should be closely monitored for side effects, particularly hypertension and diabetes mellitus.

Systemic antibiotics are often necessary due to secondary bacterial infections, especially with *Staphylococcus aureus*. Penicillin and erythromycin are safe to use in pregnancy; penicillinase-resistant penicillins are recommended for skin infections. Topical antibiotics, such as bacitracin or neomycin, are sometimes used, but they may cause skin sensitization. Mupirocin seems to be less sensitizing, but it is more expensive. Systemic antihistamines, such as hydroxyzine, diphenhydramine, chlorpheniramine, and promethazine, are often required for pruritus, and are also safe when used in pregnancy. However, newer antihistamines, such as terfenadine and cetirizine, should be avoided[3].

Both ultraviolet B (UVB) irradiation and photochemotherapy using psoralens with long-wave ultraviolet irradiation (PUVA) may be useful adjuncts in treating chronic atopic eczema. However, PUVA should not be used as a first-line treatment because of its potential adverse effects on the fetus. Occasionally, immunosuppressive agents, such as azathioprine and cyclosporin A, are required for severe eczema. These drugs should only be used with great caution during pregnancy. There is a tendency for atopic dermatitis to improve in pregnancy, though in some patients it can be exacerbated[6].

NIPPLE ECZEMA

Breastfeeding can sometimes be a problem because of nipple eczema (**8.2**). Painful fissures may develop and become secondarily infected with bacteria, particularly *S. aureus*. Anatomic features, such as relatively flat nipples, contribute to the development of this problem. Nipple eczema is treated with frequent moisturizers and a topical corticosteroid of mild potency, such as hydrocortisone. A topical corticosteroid combined with a topical antibiotic, such as fucidin H, is useful for eczema that has become infected by bacteria. A systemic antibiotic, such as erythromycin, may then be required.

HAND ECZEMA

Hand eczema may be exacerbated during the puerperium because of the constant exposure to irritants used in providing care for young children (**8.3**). Once the skin barrier has been broken, only minor re-exposure to the irritant is needed to keep the eczema active. Treatment is prophylactic and aimed at pro-

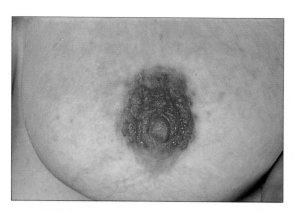

8.2 Nipple eczema. Dry, scaly, erythematous areas on nipple with painful fissures.

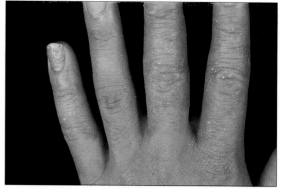

8.3 Hand eczema. Erythematous scaly areas on the dorsal and lateral aspects of the fingers. Painful fissures develop which may become secondarily infected with bacteria. There is horizontal ridging of involved nails.

tecting the hands from all skin irritants by using rubber gloves.

Topical corticosteroids of moderate potency (Class 4 or 5), such as betamethasone valerate, 0.1% cream, are needed, and emollients should be applied frequently. Hand eczema may appear for the first time in women not previously affected – atopic patients are particularly susceptible.

PSORIASIS

Psoriasis affects 1.5–2% of the general population. It is an inflammatory disorder characterized by red scaly plaques on the skin. The nails are often involved and about 7% of patients have an associated seronegative inflammatory arthritis which may be debilitating. Local injuries to the skin, such as cuts, burns or other skin infections, often lead to localized psoriasis at the site of injury (Koebner phenomenon).

TYPES OF PSORIASIS

In *plaque-type psoriasis*, the commonest form of psoriasis, there are well-demarcated erythematous plaques with adherent silver scales on the surface. The lesions are most common on the extensor surfaces of the elbows and knees, the sacral area (**8.4**),

and the scalp (**8.5**). The groin may also be involved, as described in *Chapter 13*.

Guttate (drop-like) *psoriasis* is characterized by scattered pink papules, which are of uniform size and flare in crops mainly on the trunk (**8.6**) and proximal extremities. It often follows an upper respiratory infection, especially with streptococci. In *erythrodermic psoriasis*, the skin is red with a fine desquamative scale present, often over its entire surface. There are

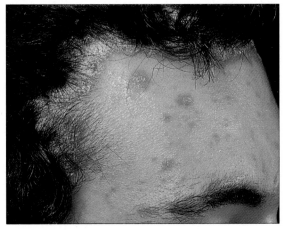

8.5 Psoriasis affecting scalp. Thick scales on scalp and hairline and smaller plaques on forehead.

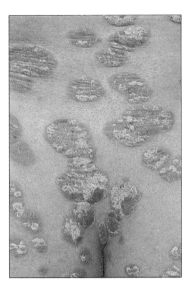

8.4 Plaque-type psoriasis. Chronic well-defined slightly raised erythematous plaques, covered by a silver scale, are present, especially over the buttocks and extensor surfaces.

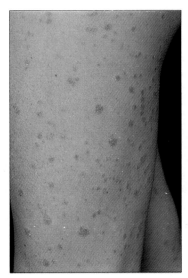

8.6 Guttate psoriasis. Small drop-like lesions occur in a shower-like distribution over the trunk and limbs, as shown here on the leg. The eruption occurs suddenly, often after a throat infection, and usually has a good prognosis.

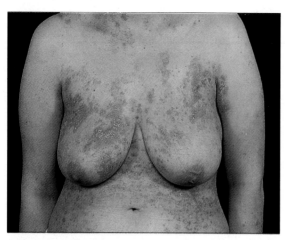

8.7 Generalized pustular psoriasis of von Zumbusch. The skin is fiery red and sore with sheets of small sterile pustules erupting on the trunk.

several forms of *pustular psoriasis*, in which small sterile pustules appear either on pre-existing plaques or *de novo* on normal skin. Most patients with pustular psoriasis have had psoriasis previously. *Generalized pustular psoriasis* (von Zumbusch) may be life-threatening and treatment is urgently required (**8.7**). Fever, arthralgias and leukocytosis often accompany the eruption. Pustular psoriasis of the palms and soles (*palmoplantar pustulosis*) consists of sterile itchy pustules on an erythematosquamous background.

MANAGEMENT

The treatment of psoriasis ranges from the application of mild tar products to the use of immunosuppressive agents. The location of lesions is important in selecting appropriate and effective therapy.

Drugs with direct therapeutic effects are used together with emollients, which will soften scaling, and keratolytics, such as salicylic acid, which help to remove the scale. Dithranol is the standard topical treatment for most cases of plaque psoriasis. However, it should be used with caution as it can irritate the skin and stain clothing. It is therefore essential to start with a low concentration and increase the dose gradually. Patients with fair skin do not tolerate dithranol as well as darker-skinned patients.

Coal tar ointment in concentrations up to 20% is often used, but as it is messy to apply and has a strong odor, it is not very popular with patients.

Topical calcipotriol, a vitamin D_3 metabolite, may be used for mild to moderately severe plaque psoriasis, but the total topical application should be less than 100g weekly to minimize possible hypercalcemia. Topical corticosteroids may be required in some forms of psoriasis, such as guttate psoriasis. Side effects may arise with long-term treatment, and a rapid relapse may occur on withdrawal (rebound phenomenon). Ultraviolet B and PUVA may be given as adjuncts to topical therapy, with special considerations for the pregnant patient (*see below*).

PREGNANCY

Dithranol, tar, calcipotriol and topical corticosteroids can all safely be used in pregnancy.

Ultraviolet B and PUVA
Ultraviolet B irradiation is safe in pregnancy, but the patient should be aware that UVB can increase the size and number of benign pigmented nevi. The use of PUVA may carry a risk of mutagenesis and teratogenesis, as discussed above with regard to eczema, and neither systemic nor topical (bath) PUVA should be used as a first-line treatment in pregnancy. However, a recent large study by Gunnarskog *et al.*[2] has found no increased risk of spontaneous or induced abortions nor an increased risk of congenital malformations or infant death, including in pregnancies conceived following PUVA treatment.

The study, however, found an increased number of low birth weight infants in pregnancies begun following PUVA treatment. It therefore seems possible that PUVA treatment may cause germ-cell mutations, resulting in chromosome anomalies or point mutations. Prenatal diagnosis should therefore be offered to women who become pregnant after PUVA treatment. Topical PUVA (bath PUVA) is safe to use in pregnancy.

Systemic Drugs
Systemic drugs are sometimes required to treat psoriasis. Retinoic acid (etretinate or acitretin) is highly teratogenic and should be used with caution (*see below*). Several cytotoxic drugs have been used for psoriasis, including methotrexate, hydroxyurea, and azathioprine. Methotrexate and hydroxyurea are known teratogens and must therefore be avoided in pregnancy, while azathioprine may be teratogenic (*see below*). Cyclosporin A should be used with caution in pregnancy and during breastfeeding, though the risks are not clear (*see below*)[7].

Course of Disease

Psoriasis remains unaltered during about 40% of pregnancies, is improved in a further 40%, and is worsened in 15% of pregnancies[8]. However, during the three months following delivery, 30% of cases will remain unchanged, 10% will improve, and 50% will deteriorate[8]. Pregnancy may also be a risk factor for psoriatic arthritis[9].

IMPETIGO HERPETIFORMIS

Impetigo herpetiformis is a very rare, acute, pustular form of psoriasis, which is precipitated by pregnancy. It can affect pregnant women with no prior history of psoriasis. The onset is usually in the third trimester, and the disease tends to persist until delivery but may continue thereafter.

The eruption characteristically begins in the flexures with small sterile pustules on areas of acutely inflamed skin. These then extend centrifugally onto the trunk (**8.8**) and around the umbilicus (**8.9**) or form plaques with green-yellow pustules. The eruption may advance and become widespread, involving the tongue, buccal mucosa, and sometimes the esophagus. Constitutional symptoms are common, including fever, delirium, vomiting, diarrhea and tetany due to hypocalcemia. Death may occur as a result of cardiac or renal failure.

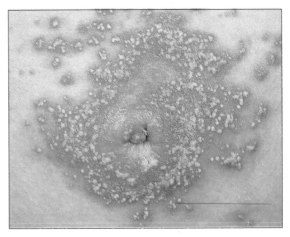

8.9 Impetigo herpetiformis. Sterile pustules around the umbilicus.

The main obstetric problem in impetigo herpetiformis is placental insufficiency, with an increased risk of stillbirth, neonatal death, and fetal abnormalities[10]. The disease characteristically recurs with each pregnancy, with earlier onset and increased morbidity[10]. Between pregnancies, patients are free of the disorder and have no manifestations of psoriasis. The disease may also be exacerbated by oral contraceptives[11]. Corticosteroids are the treatment of choice for impetigo herpetiformis, but the results are generally unsatisfactory. In severe cases, termination of pregnancy is required; the impetigo herpetiformis will usually resolve soon afterwards.

ACNE VULGARIS

Although acne may improve in pregnancy, it is occasionally exacerbated. This usually causes management problems, as most antiacne drugs are contraindicated during pregnancy. However, topical antiacne therapy, other than topical retinoic acid, does not seem to be teratogenic.

MANAGEMENT

The treatment of acne depends on the type of acne involved. If only comedones are present, a keratolytic agent such as benzoyl peroxide (2.5–10% cream, lotion or gel) or azaleic acid cream should be used to

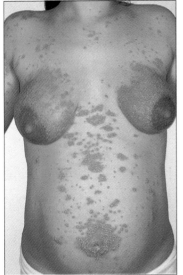

8.8 Impetigo herpetiformis. Sterile pustules develop on acutely inflamed skin which coalesce together on the trunk.

remove the surface keratin and unplug the follicular openings. These drugs are safe to use in pregnancy. Topical retinoic acid has been reported as causing multiple congenital defects in one patient[12] and ear deformities in another[13]. Ultraviolet light has an effect similar to that of topical keratolytics, but should be avoided in pregnancy.

Antibiotics

Long-term antibiotic therapy is usually required for inflammatory lesions with papules, pustules or nodules. However, acne is slow to improve and beneficial effects will not usually be seen for at least two to three months, with gradual improvement after 6–12 months of therapy. Maintenance treatment must be continued until the acne improves. Oral erythromycin is usually safe in pregnancy and is given at a dose of 250–500mg twice daily.

Topical antibiotics are almost as effective as systemic antibiotics, but they may lead to the selection of resistant bacteria on the skin surface and to contact-allergic eczema. However, as there is negligible systemic absorption, this approach is safe in pregnancy. Examples include topical clindamycin (Dalacin-T, Cleocin-T), erythromycin (Steimycin, Erygel, Erycettes, Benzamycin, and Zineryt which contains zinc in addition to erythromycin to help reduce bacterial resistance and make it more effective), and tetracycline (Topicycline – which is no longer available in the USA). These topical preparations should be applied once or twice daily to the face and/or upper trunk.

Systemic Drugs

Systemic antiandrogens and isotretinoin (Accutane, Roaccutane) are completely contraindicated in pregnancy. Vitamin A derivatives, such as oral isotretinoin, etretinate, and the newer drug acitretin, are all potent teratogens, and must not be used by those who are pregnant or who may become pregnant during the course of treatment. The most common teratogenic effects include nervous system anomalies, ear and eye deformities, cleft palate, renal and urogenital tract abnormalities, skeletal malformations, and toxic hepatocellular damage.

Although isotretinoin is rapidly cleared and is not stored in tissue, pregnancy should be avoided until two months after the drug has been discontinued. However, etretinate and its metabolite, acitretin, are potential hazards for two years after therapy has been stopped because of their very slow elimination from the body.

HIDRADENITIS SUPPURATIVA

Hidradenitis suppurativa is a chronic cutaneous disease, caused by the occlusion and rupture of follicular units, in which the resulting inflammatory response may secondarily involve the apocrine glands. Recurrent lesions develop in the axillae (**8.10**), groin, and perineal areas, with the formation of abscesses, and with draining sinuses and progressive scarring.

In extreme cases, the entire vulva may be affected over many years, resulting in gross scarring and deformity; this is often associated with substantial psychosexual problems. It often remits during pregnancy due to reduced apocrine gland activity[14].

MANAGEMENT

Management often involves the use of long-term systemic antibiotics, such as erythromycin or tetracycline. However, tetracycline should be stopped prior to a planned pregnancy. If antibiotics are unsuccessful, alternatives include oral acitretin (which must also not be used in pregnancy) or surgery where all the apocrine glands in the affected areas are excised. More recently, the carbon dioxide laser has been used to treat this condition with considerable success[15]. Although repeat treatments may be necessary, the clearance rates and the cosmetic results are excellent.

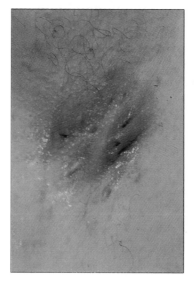

8.10 Hidradenitis suppurativa. Indolent painful pustules and nodules with sinus and scar formation in the axilla.

FOX-FORDYCE DISEASE

This is an uncommon, chronic eruption of apocrine gland-bearing skin caused by the blockage and intra-epidermal rupture of apocrine ducts. It mainly affects the axillary (**8.11**) and pubic regions, though other areas, such as the areolae, periumbilical region, and the perineum, are also sometimes involved. Itching can be intense and this may precede the formation of typical skin-colored follicular papules. The condition usually improves in pregnancy.

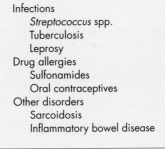

Infections
    Streptococcus spp.
    Tuberculosis
    Leprosy
Drug allergies
    Sulfonamides
    Oral contraceptives
Other disorders
    Sarcoidosis
    Inflammatory bowel disease

Table 8.1 Underlying Conditions of Erythema Nodosum.

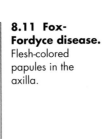

8.11 Fox-Fordyce disease. Flesh-colored papules in the axilla.

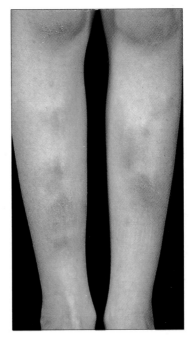

8.12 Erythema nodosum. Large painful shiny erythematous plaques on anterior aspect of lower leg. The lesions are initially bright red in color and then become purple and fade like a bruise.

ERYTHEMA NODOSUM

Erythema nodosum is a reactive inflammation of the subcutaneous fat, which is secondary to a wide variety of underlying conditions (**Table 8.1**). It can also occur in pregnancy *de novo*[16]. It presents with the sudden onset of ill-defined, tender, erythematous nodules or plaques, distributed symmetrically over the anterior legs (**8.12**). Lesions may also develop over the calves, arms, trunk, and face. Fever, malaise, and arthralgias may precede or accompany the eruption. Lesions usually resolve in six to eight weeks.

MANAGEMENT

Treatment is supportive, and includes bed-rest and mild analgesics such as paracetamol. Non-steroidal anti-inflammatory agents should not be used in pregnancy, especially in the third trimester. This is because they may constrict the ductus arteriosus *in utero*, or inhibit or prolong labor by inhibiting prostaglandin synthetase. Systemic corticosteroids, if not contra-indicated by an underlying infectious disease, are necessary in some cases. Treatment of the underlying disease or removal of the inciting drugs is essential.

INFECTIONS

During normal pregnancy, cell-mediated immunity is impaired[17]. Certain infections may appear for the first time, may occur more frequently, or may become more severe (*see also Chapter 10*).

VARICELLA-ZOSTER

Varicella (Chickenpox)

Rarely, the varicella-zoster virus (VZV) can infect pregnant women. Primary maternal infection (varicella, chickenpox) may occasionally result in severe complications, including obstetric complications such as premature labor. Pneumonia occurs in about 14% of women affected with varicella, of which 3% may die[18]. The classic congenital varicella syndrome occasionally develops if primary maternal varicella occurs during the first trimester.

Herpes Zoster (Shingles)

Recurrence of VZV as herpes zoster (shingles) is much more common in adults than primary varicella infections and does not appear to cause complications during pregnancy or adverse fetal effects.

Treatment

There are presently no data on the use of acyclovir in pregnant women with varicella or herpes zoster, though the drug is thought to have potential benefit[19]. Zoster immunoglobulin and plasma have been recommended for neonates born to infected mothers, but there are no data to suggest they are helpful in susceptible or infected pregnant women.

ACQUIRED IMMUNODEFICIENCY SYNDROME (AIDS)

There have been many pregnancies in women infected by human immunodeficiency virus (HIV). The infection is often not clinically apparent, with the first manifestation being the development of acquired immunodeficiency syndrome (AIDS) in a child after delivery. However, pregnancy appears to accelerate the development of AIDS symptoms in asymptomatic HIV-positive patients[20,21]. Opportunistic infections, such as *Pneumocystis carinii* pneumonia[22] and listeriosis[23], carry a worse prognosis in a pregnant woman than in a non-pregnant AIDS patient (almost 100% versus 30% mortality respectively). Disseminated

Kaposi's sarcoma has been reported in pregnant women with AIDS[24]. The effects of AIDS on the fetus can be devastating with the fullblown syndrome developing in a high percentage of infants, usually within 16 months of birth. Intrauterine growth retardation and prematurity have also been reported[18]. Viral infections such as herpes simplex and condylomata are likely to deteriorate with the progression of AIDS. As might be expected, lesions may become extensive in pregnant AIDS patients. Severe seborrheic dermatitis and/or recalcitrant thrush or vulvovaginal candidosis should raise the suspicion of possible HIV disease in a pregnant woman.

LEPROSY

More than one-third of patients with leprosy will experience an exacerbation of their disease during pregnancy or in the first six months following delivery[25]. This can be expressed by:
- The appearance of new lesions;
- The extension of established lesions;
- The development of erythema in tuberculoid lesions (**8.13**);
- A rise in the bacillary concentration in split-skin smears;
- A rise in the proportion of viable bacilli in smears.

Leprosy rendered quiescent by chemotherapy may relapse, and subclinical disease may become apparent for the first time during pregnancy.

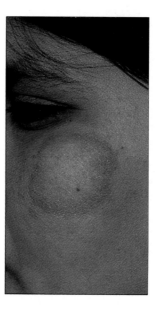

8.13 Tuberculoid leprosy. Anesthetic, annular erythematous plaque on cheek.

Lepra Reactions

Type 1 and type 2 lepra reactions become more common during pregnancy, especially in the first trimester and early postpartum period. A high percentage of patients with type 2 reactions have *erythema nodosum leprosum*, with painful red nodules that may suppurate or ulcerate almost continually from the third trimester until 15 months postpartum[26] (**8.14**). During pregnancy, the lepra reaction is most commonly expressed as skin involvement, whereas nerve involvement is the most frequent manifestation postpartum. Low birth weights and small placentae have been reported and may account for the high incidence of infant mortality[27].

Management

The treatment of leprosy must be modified in pregnancy. Dapsone, 100mg daily, is probably safe, but thalidomide is totally contraindicated since it is teratogenic, and even clofazimine has been associated with unexplained fetal deaths[28]. Lepra reactions should be treated with prednisone, 40–60mg daily, for about two weeks, followed by a steady reduction in dose. The depressed immune status of the patient may cause an increase in drug resistance. Whenever possible, before they become pregnant, patients should be told that there is a significant risk their condition will deteriorate during pregnancy. Ideally, pregnancies should be planned when the leprosy is well controlled.

BULLOUS DISORDERS

PEMPHIGUS

Pemphigus is an uncommon autoimmune bullous dermatosis, which may develop or worsen during pregnancy and be transmitted to the fetus. It is important that obstetricians and dermatologists maintain close antenatal and postnatal care of the mother and child. Pemphigus is caused by an autoantibody directed against epidermal antigens. Flaccid blisters of the skin (**8.15**) and mucous membranes develop, and are often widespread. The blisters rapidly rupture, leading to generalized erosions, crusting, and often secondary bacterial infections.

The presentation of pemphigus during pregnancy is extremely rare, though pregnancy has been reported to precipitate or aggravate the disease[29]. Exacerbations usually occur in the first or second trimester, and in most cases the disease continues chronically

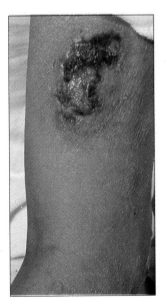

8.14 Erythema nodosum leprosum.
Ulcerating erythema nodosum leprosum on the upper arm of a Bangladeshi patient.

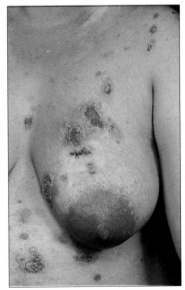

8.15 Pemphigus vulgaris.
Superficial, flaccid blisters on upper trunk easily rupture leaving erosions. Blisters may become secondarily infected with bacteria and become crusted.

postpartum. It has been suggested that the improvement seen in pemphigus in the third trimester is due to a rising endogenous cortisol production and consequent immunosuppression. The clinical presentation of pemphigus can be very similar to that of pemphigoid gestationis (PG), and so skin biopsy with immunofluorescence studies is required for an accurate diagnosis[18] (*see also Chapter 17, p. 130*).

Management

Pemphigus during pregnancy is usually treated with high doses of prednisone. *Steroid* doses as high as 100mg prednisone daily may be required for initial control, with dose tapering thereafter. A potent topical corticosteroid cream, such as 0.05% clobetasol propionate, can be applied directly to lesions.

Immunosuppressants, such as cyclophosphamide, azathioprine, methotrexate, and gold, are best avoided. Azathioprine has not been associated with teratogenicity, but it could theoretically affect the immune system of the fetus or neonate. It is not recommended in breastfeeding mothers. Methotrexate is a potent teratogen, particularly if taken during the first trimester, causing multiple skeletal and neurologic defects and cleft palate. Although it is secreted in relatively low concentrations in breast milk, breastfeeding is usually not recommended. There is little data on the safety of cyclosporin A in pregnant dermatology patients. A study of pregnant women taking cyclosporin A following organ transplantation suggests a low risk of teratogenic effects. As cyclosporin A passes into breast milk, there is therefore a potential risk of hypertension, nephrotoxicity, and malignancy in breastfed neonates. Cyclophosphamide is teratogen leading to skeletal defects and dysmorphic features.

Pemphigus antibody titers may help in assessing disease activity and planning effective treatment. If high antibody titers occur, transplacental transfer of pemphigus antibody and transient fetal pemphigus is probably more likely[30]. Plasmapheresis has been used but there is a risk of a rebound increase in circulating levels of pemphigus antibody. There appears to be, therefore, a need for continued plasmapheresis after delivery, with immunosuppressant adjunctive treatment (e.g. azathioprine) making this an option of last resort.

Maternal and Fetal Mortality and Morbidity

Severe cases of disseminated cutaneous disease have been associated with fetal death. Cases of well-controlled or mild disease are not usually associated with a significant risk of maternal and fetal morbidity or mortality. The mode of delivery needs careful consideration in each case. The trauma of vaginal delivery may result in the extension and worsening of erosions, while problems with wound healing in patients on long-term steroid therapy make cesarean section less attractive.

Neonatal Pemphigus

Neonatal pemphigus results from transplacental transmission of maternal pemphigus IgG autoantibody. Active pemphigus during pregnancy does not necessarily result in neonatal pemphigus. Most neonates who develop blisters require no therapy, as the blisters usually heal spontaneously within two to three weeks[30]. Breastfeeding is not absolutely contraindicated, though local blister formation may occur with the potential risk of passive transfer of antibody to the infant.

DERMATITIS HERPETIFORMIS

Dermatitis herpetiformis is an autoimmune vesicular disorder characterized by grouped, intensely pruritic vesicles, which are symmetrically distributed over the elbows, knees, buttocks, shoulders and scalp (**8.16**). There is usually histologic and/or symptomatic evidence of gluten-sensitive enteropathy. The

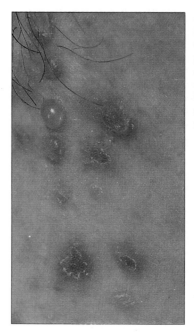

8.16 Dermatitis herpetiformis. Grouped, itchy, polymorphic lesions on extremities, such as axillae, as shown here. Vesicles are excoriated leaving urticarial papules.

characteristic immunofluorescence feature of this disease is the presence of granular deposits of IgA in the upper papillary dermis.

Management

Dapsone administration – the treatment of choice – produces dramatic relief from pruritus within 24 hours and stops new lesion formation within 72 hours. Dapsone is probably safe in pregnancy[2,31]. Most patients respond to an initial dose of 100mg daily. Those intolerant of dapsone should be tried on sulfapyridine, 1–2g daily. As dapsone may produce severe hemolysis in patients with glucose-6-phosphate dehydrogenase deficiency, patients should be screened before dapsone therapy is instituted.

Ideally, patients with dermatitis herpetiformis should adhere to a strict gluten-free diet, preferably for 6–12 months, before conception. This may obviate the need for dapsone during pregnancy. As dapsone is secreted in breastmilk and produces hemolytic anemia in infants, patients taking dapsone should be discouraged from breastfeeding.

LINEAR IgA DISEASE

This is a rare, acquired, subepidermal blistering disorder. It has been defined on the basis of its unique immunopathologic finding of linear deposits of IgA along the cutaneous basement membrane. It clinically resembles dermatitis herpetiformis, but sometimes lesions similar to bullous pemphigoid develop on the trunk and limbs. Unlike dermatitis herpetiformis, there is no associated gluten-sensitive enteropathy.

Linear IgA disease may improve in pregnancy but a relapse may be seen postpartum[32]. The disease does not appear to affect fetal outcome adversely. Treatment is similar to that of dermatitis herpetiformis, with dapsone or sulfapyridine, but some patients may need a combination of dapsone and prednisone (*see also Chapter 17*).

PORPHYRIA CUTANEA TARDA

Porphyria cutanea tarda (PCT) is the most common type of porphyria and occurs in both autosomal-dominant and acquired forms. The disorder is due to a defect in uroporphyrinogen decarboxylase activity. This results in a characteristic increase of uroporphyrin and 7-carboxyporphyrin in the urine, and increased isocoproporphyrin in the stool. Patients present with skin fragility, erosions, vesicles, bullae, and milia on sun-exposed areas, especially the dorsum of the hands (**8.17**) and forearms. Other cutaneous changes include facial hypertrichosis, periorbital hyperpigmentation, scarring alopecia, and dystrophic calcification with ulceration.

Pregnancy

Although PCT is known to be affected adversely by estrogen, iron, and alcohol, there are conflicting reports about the effects of pregnancy. Case reports of patients whose illness was not exacerbated by pregnancy have led to speculation that endogenous estrogens may be less harmful than exogenous compounds[33]. However, other cases show findings of clinical and biochemical deterioration of disease, with increases in plasma and urine porphyrins during pregnancy[34,35].

Management

The avoidance of sunlight and use of an opaque sun block, such as zinc oxide, are helpful. Venesection or phlebotomy, with careful monitoring of hematocrit, has been used successfully to treat porphyria cutanea tarda during pregnancy. In this procedure, 500ml of blood is removed weekly or twice weekly until the hemoglobin level has fallen to 10–11g/dl or serum iron to 50–60mg/dl.

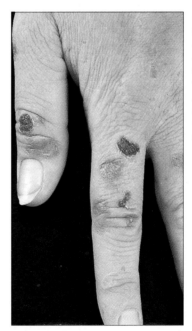

8.17 Porphyria cutanea tarda. Sun-exposed areas, such as the dorsum of the hand and fingers, are most severely affected. Minimal trauma results in erosions and blisters.

Chloroquine is contraindicated in pregnancy because of its teratogenicity; it causes multiple defects in the fetus, including neurosensory hearing loss, mental retardation, and neonatal convulsions. Other less commonly applied therapies, such as cholestyramine, activated charcoal, and intravenous deferoxamine administration, are also contraindicated in pregnancy.

ERYTHEMA MULTIFORME

This disorder is characterized by acute, self-limiting, but often recurrent episodes of erythematous maculopapular lesions, which may develop into classical target or iris lesions, or may blister. The lesions are typically distributed symmetrically on the extremities, especially the hands (**8.18**), and on the extensor aspects of the forearms and legs. The frequency of mucosal involvement varies widely between 25% and 60%, with affected organs including the mouth, eyes, pharynx, esophagus, genitalia, and anus. Severe cases (Stevens–Johnson syndrome) may develop significant complications, such as visual impairment secondary to keratitis with conjunctival scarring (**8.19**).

There are several causes of erythema multiforme, such as herpes simplex or mycoplasmal infections, and sensitivity to drugs, especially to long-acting sulfonamides. Pregnancy may also cause erythema multiforme, and vaginal stenosis has been described in severe Stevens–Johnson syndrome in pregnancy[36]. Systemic corticosteroids, such as prednisone, 30–40mg daily, are sometimes required, particularly in Stevens–Johnson syndrome. The dose should be gradually reduced after a few days.

NEOPLASIA

Basal cell epithelioma and *squamous cell carcinoma* are both very rare in pregnancy, as they tend to be disorders of the elderly population. *Gorlin syndrome* (basal cell nevus syndrome) is a rare autosomal-dominant inherited condition, in which numerous basal cell carcinomas develop in a much younger age group; there are few reports in pregnant women. The disorder certainly does not appear to affect this group specifically.

BENIGN MELANOCYTIC NEVI

It is known that pre-existing benign pigmented nevi may temporarily darken during pregnancy and increase in number and size (**8.20**). However, there is no evidence that pregnancy induces malignant transformation of pre-existing nevi.

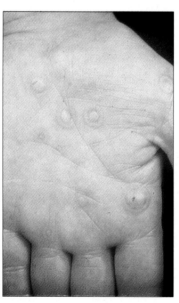

8.18 Erythema multiforme. Well-circumscribed erythematous lesions occur on the hands, as shown here, and feet. The central area of the lesion is more involved than the periphery so it appears like a target. Blisters may develop in the center of the lesions.

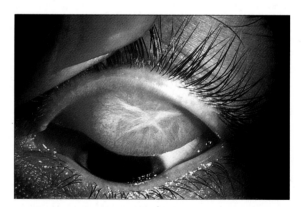

8.19 Stevens–Johnson syndrome. Severe blistering and ulceration of the conjunctiva results in corneal scarring.

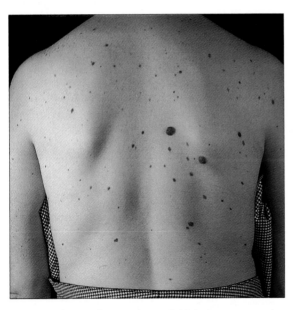

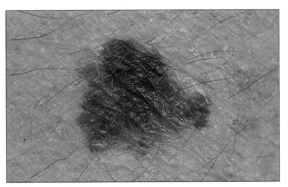

8.21 Superficial malignant melanoma. The pigmented lesion is a slightly raised plaque with an irregular outline and irregular pigmentation.

8.20 Benign melanocytic nevi. Multiple nevi on trunk have evenly distributed pigment and each nevus has a regular outline.

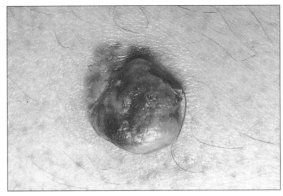

8.22 Nodular malignant melanoma. A nodule has developed in the center of an irregularly outlined pigmented lesion. The nodule itself appears to be relatively amelanotic.

MALIGNANT MELANOMA

The influence of pregnancy on the prognosis of malignant melanoma (**8.21, 8.22**) is controversial[37–39]. Many early observations suggested a link between hormones and malignant melanoma, but these have been disputed, and the suspected adverse effect of pregnancy on malignant melanoma has not been confirmed. Mackie *et al.* have published a large study which suggests that malignant melanoma developing during pregnancy has a slightly worse prognosis. However, pregnancy following excision of a tumor does not appear to affect prognosis, which continues to be determined mainly by tumor thickness[40]. Transplacental transmission of melanoma to the fetus is extremely rare, and maternal melanoma usually has no adverse effects on the fetus[37].

Management

Treatment for melanoma in pregnant women is no different to treatment in other patients. Surgical excision of primary lesions and clinically involved lymph nodes should be performed. Therapeutic termination in a woman who has a concurrent malignant melanoma and pregnancy has shown no benefit in preventing fetal metastasis or inducing maternal

tumor regression[37]. When melanoma occurs during pregnancy, a clinical and histologic examination of the placenta should be performed postpartum, as the possibility of transmission of transplacental metastatic disease to the fetus does exist[18].

Timing of Pregnancy

Women from whom malignant melanomas have been excised should be counselled about future pregnancies. Mackie *et al.* have observed that 83% of patients with metastatic disease present within two years after the initial diagnosis of their primary malignant melanoma. Women should therefore be recommended to delay pregnancy by at least two years after diagnosis[40]. Generally, women with melanoma should be advised about pregnancy on the basis of thickness and site of tumor and evidence of vascular spread, not hormonal status[40].

CUTANEOUS T-CELL LYMPHOMA

Cutaneous T-cell lymphoma (CTCL) or mycosis fungoides is a chronic, slowly evolving, T-cell lymphoma involving mainly the skin. The earliest lesions are flat, erythematous, slightly scaly patches, which gradually thicken to form plaques. Sometimes tumors may develop. Pregnancy may exacerbate the disease[41].

Early lesions may respond to potent topical steroids and UVB, but PUVA should be avoided, if possible, because of the potential teratogenic effects of methoxypsoralen. Therapy with cytotoxic agents is generally contraindicated during pregnancy, especially in the first trimester.

MISCELLANEOUS CONDITIONS

SARCOIDOSIS

Sarcoidosis is a multisystem, granulomatous disorder of unknown etiology, which most commonly affects young adults in their reproductive years. Approximately 0.02–0.06% of pregnant women have sarcoidosis[42]. There are both specific and non-specific cutaneous lesions associated with sarcoidosis. Specific lesions include papules, nodules (**8.23**), plaques (lupus pernio) (**8.24**), ichthyotic scaling, hypopigmentation, atrophy, ulcers, and scar infiltration. The non-specific lesions are not actually granulomas, but skin changes which are characteristically associated with sarcoidosis – the most common of which is erythema nodosum.

Pregnancy

Active sarcoidosis usually improves during pregnancy and relapses postpartum. In cases of already inactive disease, the condition remains inactive[43]. The positive effects of pregnancy on sarcoidosis may be due to an increased amount of circulating free cortisol, and the postpartum relapse may represent a rebound phenomenon, as is usually seen after cessation of corticosteroid therapy. Improvement in some pregnant patients with sarcoidosis might be related to spontaneous resolution of the disease.

The frequency of abortions, obstetric complications, or congenital abnormalities is not increased by the presence of sarcoidosis[43]. Generally, the obstetric management of pregnancy, labor, and delivery does not differ from that for a normal patient. In some

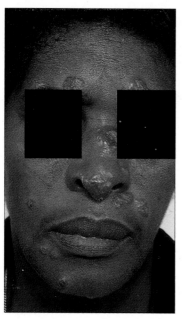

8.23 Sarcoidosis. Annular, pigmented plaques on the face. Nasal infiltration may be extremely disfiguring and difficult to treat. In West Indians, red-brown nodules are especially common around the nose.

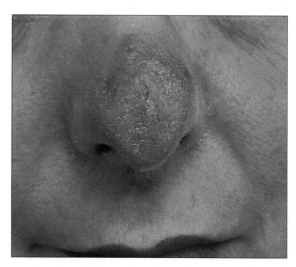

8.24 Lupus pernio. Thickened purple plaques occur on the nose and are caused by granulomatous involvement of the dermis and subcutaneous fat.

cases, however, such as those with advanced pulmonary disease or extrapulmonary lesions, exacerbations may occur and patients should be followed carefully. Disease activity should be carefully assessed soon after delivery in all patients who have, or have had, sarcoidosis[43].

ACRODERMATITIS ENTEROPATHICA

This is a rare autosomal-recessive condition with reduced serum zinc levels. Acquired zinc deficiency can occur in patients with an inadequate intake of zinc, such as those receiving long-term parenteral nutrition without zinc supplementation, those who have zinc malabsorption, and those with increased losses of zinc. It is characterized by dermatitis, diarrhea and alopecia. The dermatitis is vesiculobullous and eczematous, and develops on the acral areas of the extremities and periorificial sites, such as the mouth, anus, and genital areas. Paronychia and scalp alopecia are seen.

Acrodermatitis enteropathica flares during pregnancy, with a further decrease in serum zinc concentration[44]. This fall in zinc level is not entirely due to increased fetal demands, because zinc levels also decrease and the disease flares with oral contraceptive use[18]. Estrogens must therefore have an important primary role[44].

The skin eruption may resemble impetigo herpetiformis or pemphigoid gestationis. Having first appeared in childhood, the skin disease reappears early during pregnancy, progressively worsens until delivery, and then spontaneously clears postpartum.

Most pregnancies have produced normal offspring[18]. Zinc supplementation (e.g. zinc sulfate, 200mg three times daily) to maintain normal serum zinc levels seems to be effective in preventing adverse fetal effects.

NEUROFIBROMAS

During pregnancy, the skin lesions of neurofibromatosis may appear for the first time, or may increase in both size and number. Large, plexiform, neurofibromas may enlarge (**8.25**) and then hemorrhage into the core of the tumor. In most cases, the lesions regress postpartum. Of greater importance is the effect of pregnancy on the vascular system of patients with neurofibromatosis. Major blood vessels may

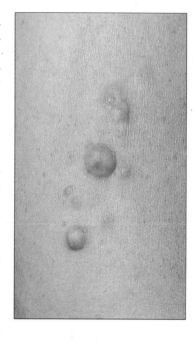

8.25 Neurofibromatosis. Large neurofibromas have developed on the upper arm.

rupture and hypertension may occur[45]. Genetic counselling is mandatory because of the disabilities that may be precipitated by pregnancy and because of the rare possible deformities associated with neurofibromatosis, an autosomal-dominant disorder. Elective termination of pregnancy may be necessary in severely affected patients.

CONCLUSION

Obstetricians and dermatologists working together should be able to recognize and manage skin diseases in pregnant women. They should be aware of the often modified expression of disease in this special group of patients, and should also realize that therapeutic options are inevitably altered by the pregnant condition. It is important that patients with inherited disorders are counselled about the genetic nature of their condition, and if necessary the dermatologist and geneticist should offer counselling before conception.

REFERENCES

1 Reed, B. R. Pregnancy, drugs and the dermatologist. *Curr. Probs Dermatol.* 1994; VI (2):29–80.

2 Stockton, D. L. and Paller, A. S. Drug administration to the pregnant or lactating woman: a reference guide for dermatologists. *J. Am. Acad. Dermatol.* 1990; **23**: 87–103.

3 Jurecka, W. and Gebhart, W. Drug prescribing during pregnancy. *Semin. Dermatol.* 1989; **8**: 30–39.

4 Gunnarskog, J. G., Kallen, A. J. B., Lindelof, B. G., *et al.* Psoralen photochemotherapy (PUVA) and pregnancy. *Arch. Dermatol.* 1993; **129**: 320–323.

5 Cockburn, I., Krupp, P., and Monka, C. Present experience of Sandimmun in pregnancy. *Transplant. Proc.* 1989; **21**: 3730–3732.

6 Kemmett, D. and Tidman, M. J. The influence of the menstrual cycle and pregnancy on atopic dermatitis. *Br. J. Dermatol.* 1991; **125**: 59–61.

7 Wright, S., Glover, M., and Baker, H. Psoriasis, cyclosporin, and pregnancy. *Arch. Dermatol.* 1991; **127**: 426.

8 Dunna, S. F. and Findlay, A. Y. Psoriasis: improvement during and worsening after pregnancy. *Br. J. Dermatol.* 1989; **120**: 584.

9 McHugh, N. J. and Laurent, M. R. The effect of pregnancy on the onset of psoriatic arthritis. *Br. J. Rheumatol.* 1989; **28**: 50–52.

10 Lotem, M., Katzenelson, V., Rotem, A., *et al.* Impetigo herpetiformis: a variant of pustular psoriasis or a separate entity? *J. Am. Acad. Dermatol.* 1989; **20**: 338–341.

11 Oumeish, O. Y., Farraj, S. E., and Bataineh, A. S. Some aspects of impetigo herpetiformis. *Arch. Dermatol.* 1982; **118**: 103–105.

12 Lipson, A. H., Collins, F., and Webster, W. S. Multiple congenital defects associated with maternal use of topical tretinoin. *Lancet* 1993; **341**: 1352–1353.

13 Camera, G. and Pregliasco, P. Ear malformation in baby born to mother using tretinoin cream. *Lancet* 1992; **339**: 687.

14 Graham–Brown, R. A. C. and Ebling, F. J. G. The ages of man and their dermatoses. In: Champion, R. H., Burton, J. L., and Ebling, F. J. G. (eds.) *Textbook of Dermatology.* Oxford: Blackwell, 1992, p.2890.

15 Dalyrumple, J.C. and Monaghan, J.M. Treatment of hidradenitis suppurativa with the carbon dioxide laser. *Br. J. Surg.* 1987; **74**: 420.

16 Bartelsmeyer, J. A. and Petrie, R. H. Erythema nodosum, estrogens, and pregnancy. *Clin. Obstet. Gynecol.* 1990; **33**: 777–781.

17 Weinberg, E. D. Pregnancy-associated depression of cell-mediated immunity. *Rev. Infect. Dis.* 1984; **5**: 814–831.

18 Winton, G. B. Skin diseases aggravated by pregnancy. *J. Am. Acad. Dermatol.* 1989; **20**: 1–13.

19 Rothe, M. J., *et al.* Oral acyclovir therapy for varicella and zoster infections in pediatric and pregnant patients. A brief review. *Ped. Dermatol.* 1991; **8**: 236.

20 Minkoff, H., Nanda, D., Menez, R., *et al.* Pregnancies resulting in infants with acquired immunodeficiency syndrome or AIDS-related complex. *Obstet. Gynecol.* 1987; **69**: 285–287.

21 Minkoff, H., Nanda, D., Menez, R., *et al.* Pregnancies resulting in infants with acquired immunodeficiency syndrome or AIDS-related complex: follow-up of mothers, children, and subsequently born siblings. *Obstet. Gynecol.* 1987; **69**: 288–291.

22 Minkoff, H., deRegt, R. H., Landesman, S., *et al.* Pneumocystis carinii pneumonia associated with acquired immunodeficiency syndrome in pregnancy: a report of three maternal deaths. *Obstet. Gynecol.* 1986; **67**: 284–287.

23 Wetli, C. V., Roldan, E. D., and Fujaco, R. M. Listerosis as a cause of maternal death: an obstetric complication of acquired immunodeficiency syndrome (AIDS). *Am. J. Obstet. Gynecol.* 1983; **147**: 7–9.

24 Rawlinson, K. F., Zubrow, A. B., Harris, M. A., *et al.* Disseminated Kaposi's sarcoma in pregnancy: a manifestation of acquired immune deficiency syndrome. *Obstet. Gynecol.* 1984: **63** (suppl.): 2–6.

25 Duncan, M. E., Pearson, J. M. H., Ridley, D. S., *et al.* Pregnancy and leprosy: the consequences of alterations of cell-mediated and humoral immunity during pregnancy and lactation. *Int. J. Lepr.* 1982; **50**: 425–435.

26 Duncan, M. E. and Pearson, J. M. H. The association of pregnancy and leprosy III. Erythema nodosum leprosum in pregnancy and lactation. *Lepr. Rev.* 1984; **55**: 129–142.

27 Duncan, M. E. Babies of mothers with leprosy have small placentae, low birthweights and grow slowly. *Br. J. Obstet. Gynaecol.* 1980; **87**: 471–479.

28 Farb, H., West, D. P., and Pedvis-Leftick, A. Clofazimine in pregnancy complicated by leprosy. *Obstet. Gynecol.* 1982; **59**: 122–123.

29 Honeyman, J. F., Eguiguren, G., Pinto, A., *et al.* Bullous dermatoses of pregnancy. *Arch. Dermatol.* 1981; **117**: 264–267.

30 Goldberg, N. S., DeFeo, C., and Kirshenbaum, N. Pemphigus vulgaris and pregnancy: risk factors and recommendations. *J. Am. Acad. Dermatol.* 1993; **28**: 877–879.

31 Kahn, G. Dapsone is safe during pregnancy (letter). *J. Am. Acad. Dermatol.* 1985; **13**: 838–839.

32 Collier, P. M., Kelly, S. E., and Wojnarowska, F. W. Linear IgA disease and pregnancy. *J. Am. Acad. Dermatol.* 1994; **30**: 407–411.

33 Marks, R. Porphyria cutanea tarda. *Arch. Dermatol.* 1982; **118**: 452.

34 Baxi, L. V., Rubeo, T. J., Katz, B., *et al.* Porphyria cutanea tarda and pregnancy. *Am. J. Obstet. Gynecol.* 1983; **146**: 333–334.

35 Rajka, G. Pregnancy and porphyria cutanea tarda. *Acta. Derm. Venereol.* (Stockh.) 1984; **64**: 444–445.

36 Graham–Brown, R. A. C., Cochrane, G. W., Swinhoe, J. R., *et al.* Vaginal stenosis due to bullous erythema multiforme (Stevens-Johnson syndrome). *Br. J. Obstet. Gynaecol.* 1981; **88**: 1156–1157.

37 Colburn, D. S., Nathanson, L., and Belilos, E. Pregnancy and malignant melanoma. *Semin. Oncol.* 1989; **16**: 377–387.

38 McManamny, D. S., Moss, A. L. H., Briggs, J. C., *et al.* Melanoma and pregnancy: a long-term follow-up. *Br. J. Obstet. Gynaecol.* 1989; **96**: 1419–1423.

39 Driscoll, M. S., Grin-Jorgensen, C. M., Grant-Kels, J. M. Does pregnancy influence the prognosis of malignant melanoma? *J. Am. Acad. Dermatol.* 1993; **29**: 619–630.

40 Mackie, R. M., Bufalino, R., Morabito, A., *et al.* Lack of effect of pregnancy on outcome of melanoma. *Lancet* 1991; i: 653–655.

41 Vonderheid, E. C., Dellatorre, D. L., and van Scott, E. J. Prolonged remission of tumor-stage mycosis fungoides by topical immunotherapy. *Arch. Dermatol.* 1981; **117**: 586–589.

42 Abarquez, C., Panda and Sharma, O. P. Sarcoidosis and pregnancy. *Sarcoidosis J.* 1990; **7**(1): 63–66.

43 Selroos, O. Sarcoidosis and pregnancy: a review with results of a retrospective survey. *J. Int. Med.* 1990; **227**(4): 221–224.

44 Bronson, D. M., Barsky, R., and Barsky, S. Acrodermatitis enteropathica: recognition at long last during a recurrence in pregnancy. *J. Am. Acad. Dermatol.* 1983; **9**: 140–144.

45 Braude, P. B. and Bolan, J. C. Neurofibromatosis and spontaneous hemothorax in pregnancy: two case reports. *Obstet. Gynecol.* 1984; **63** (suppl.): 35–38.

ACKNOWLEDGEMENTS

Figure **8.3** has been reproduced by kind permission of Dr I. R. White, St John's Institute of Dermatology, St Thomas' Hospital, London, UK. Figures **8.8** and **8.9** have been reproduced by kind permission of Dr. A. C. Pembroke, King's College Hospital, London, UK. Figure **8.14** has been reproduced by kind permission of Dr A.D.M. Bryceson, Hospital for Tropical Diseases, London, UK.

9.
Connective Tissue Diseases in Pregnancy

Neil N. M. Buchanan, Munther A. Khamashta, Sian Kerslake &
Graham R. V. Hughes

The connective tissue diseases are multisystem disorders characterized by circulating non-organ specific autoantibodies. Many of them, notably systemic lupus erythematosus (SLE) and Sjogren's syndrome, have a strong female bias (9:1), and are thought to be influenced by female sex hormones. Pregnancy, as a state of hormonal and immunologic alteration, interacts with many of these diseases in clinically significant ways.

RHEUMATOID ARTHRITIS

The activity of rheumatoid arthritis (RA) is altered significantly in pregnancy, with about 70% of mothers showing marked improvement of both joint and extra-articular features. Occasionally, however, the disease may worsen, and there are reports of RA first presenting in pregnancy. Up to 90% of mothers relapse in the first six months after delivery, with consequent problems for childcare. Active disease does not seem to alter fetal or maternal outcome.

SYSTEMIC LUPUS ERYTHEMATOSUS

Systemic lupus erythematosus is now recognized as a much more common disease worldwide than previously believed. In some countries, notably in the Far East, its prevalence has overtaken that of RA. Until

comparatively recently, it was widely regarded as a disease of uniformly poor prognosis, in which pregnancy was to be discouraged. Now, with the recognition of milder forms of the disease, and more conservative approaches to treatment, pregnancy is common in SLE patients, who are mostly aged between 16 and 45. Fertility is usually normal in SLE.

Disease flares are probably no commoner in pregnancy than in the non-pregnant state. Our own studies have found that the rate of disease flares is similar in all three trimesters, and that this rate is similar to the rate of flares in the non-pregnant state. Cutaneous flares are the most common (**9.1–9.4**), followed by joint symptoms (**9.5**).

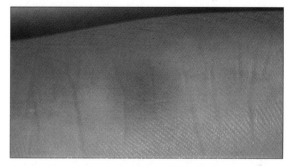

9.2 Palmar lupus vasculitis. This palmar lupus vasculitic lesion was painful.

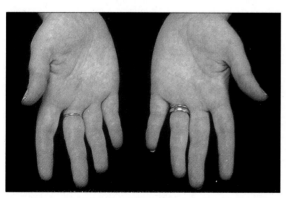

9.1 Florid erythema of the palms. Pregnancy related palmar erythema may confuse the diagnosis of lupus vasculitis.

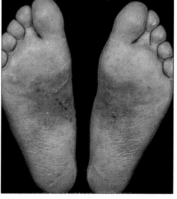

9.3 Lupus vasculitis of the soles. This young woman had marked lupus vasculitis of the soles of the feet, which had been confused with a fungal dermatosis by her family physician.

Active renal disease may be difficult to distinguish from pregnancy-associated hypertension (**Table 9.1**). Active lupus is associated with an increase in preterm deliveries and small-for-gestational-age (SGA) babies, while active renal disease may lead to more frequent fetal losses. These factors support the treatment of active lupus from the fetal, as well as from the maternal, point of view. As drugs used in connective tissue disorders are potentially hazardous, their use should be tailored to their likely efficacy and the severity of the disease process (**Table 9.2**).

Evidence of clinical lupus activity in other systems
Rising titer of antiDNA antibodies
Evidence of alternative pathway complement activation
Presence of cellular casts on urine microscopy

Table 9.1   Features Distinguishing Renal Flare in Lupus Pregnancy from Pregnancy-Associated Hypertension.

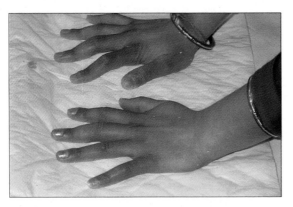

9.4   Peripheral lupus vasculitis. Vasculitic rashes in lupus pregnancy commonly affect the peripheries, especially the tips of the fingers and toes.

Drug	Relative Safety
Prednisone	High (especially in doses of 20mg daily or less)
Sulfasalazine	High
Aspirin (low doses)	High
Heparin	High (though osteoporosis is a real risk)
Gold	Caution (best avoided)
Azathioprine	Caution (probably safe)
Hydroxychloroquine	Caution (probably safe at the lower doses now used, e.g. 200mg daily)
Nifedipine	Caution
Penicillamine	Low
Methotrexate	Contraindicated in pregnancy
Cyclophosphamide	Low
Warfarin	Low (avoid in first trimester)

Table 9.2   Drug Treatment of Connective Tissue Disease in Pregnancy.

9.5   Arthritic lupus flare. After skin manifestations, an 'arthritic' flare of lupus (joint pain and swelling) is the second commonest type of flare in lupus pregnancy. Morning stiffness, a prominent symptom in this mother's case, may help to distinguish true inflammatory arthritis from periarticular and soft-tissue swelling found in normal pregnancy.

NEONATAL LUPUS ERYTHEMATOSUS

Two clinicoserologic subgroups of lupus have important implications for fetal and neonatal health. Circulating antiRo (SS-A) antibodies, often in mothers with predominantly cutaneous lupus and Sjögren's syndrome, can cross the placenta to the fetus, resulting in neonatal lupus erythematosus (NLE).

The commonest manifestation of NLE is a cutaneous eruption (**9.6**), which often begins some weeks after birth and usually resolves by about six months of age. The lesions tend to be annular, erythematous and scaly and occur over the face or other light-exposed skin. As they resolve without scarring, the only treatment needed is the avoidance of exposure to sunlight.

Congenital heart block

Congenital heart block is a rarer, more serious form of NLE, occurring in perhaps 2% of pregnancies to mothers who have circulating antiRo. Its onset at, or after, 18 weeks of gestation should be looked for using ultrasound (**9.7, 9.8**). Intrauterine treatment of heart block has been unsuccessful. However, despite significant perinatal mortality, the infants usually do well. In about 50% of cases, the child may require a pacemaker by 12 years of age. The risk of a second child being born with heart block is one in four, rising to one in two after two or more affected babies. However, it should be emphasized that, although antiRo antibodies occur in about 25% of all lupus patients, the risk of congenital heart block is small.

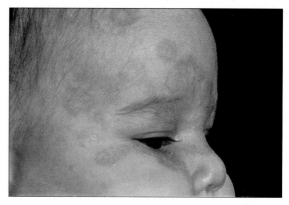

9.6 Cutaneous neonatal lupus. This baby shows the classical appearance of neonatal lupus.

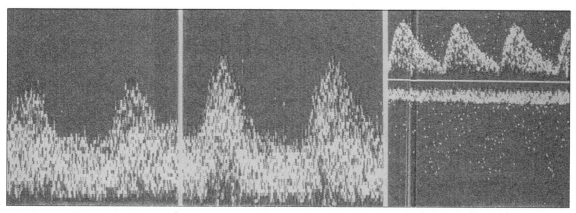

9.7 Normal fetal heartbeat. Normal Doppler blood-flow studies at 19 weeks' gestation. The left and center windows show normal right and left umbilical artery blood flows. The right-hand window shows the flow in the umbilical artery. The overall picture is of a normal fetal heart rate pattern in the umbilical artery of 140 beats per minute and normal end-diastolic blood flow.

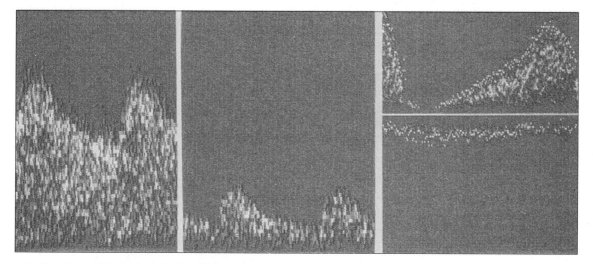

9.8 Fetal heart block. Doppler blood-flow studies detecting heart block in a fetus at 23 weeks' gestation. The fetal heart rate is 60 beats per minute, and shows complete heart block combined with absent end-diastolic flow. The infant was subsequently delivered at 34 weeks' gestation uneventfully, and is alive and well.

THE ANTIPHOSPHOLIPID SYNDROME

Ten years ago, Hughes first described a clinical syndrome associated with the presence of circulating antibodies (lupus anticoagulant) against phospholipids[1]. This syndrome consists of a tendency to recurrent venous and arterial thromboses, recurrent miscarriage, livedo reticularis (**9.9**), migraine, strokes, labile hypertension and occasional thrombocytopenia. Indolent cutaneous ulcers (**9.10**) are a rare feature of this condition. Although the antiphospholipid syndrome was first described as a feature of some lupus patients, it is now recognized as a 'primary' antiphospholipid syndrome. Recurrent miscarriage is one of the many presentations of the syndrome, and anticardiolipin screening is now carried out worldwide in obstetrics clinics, as part of the investigation of recurrent abortion.

TREATMENT

Treatment with low-dose aspirin and, where there is a history of thrombosis, with subcutaneous heparin, appears to reduce fetal mortality significantly. There is no evidence that prednisone (prednisolone) is helpful. Comparative trials are now taking place in many centers, in particular comparing aspirin and heparin regimes.

SCLERODERMA

The interactions between scleroderma and pregnancy are unclear. Although reduced fertility and increased fetal loss are suspected, they are not proven. In the third trimester, hypertension and renal failure are potential risks for the mother and can be fatal. Tight abdominal and breast skin and worsening esophagitis should be anticipated.

DERMATOMYOSITIS AND POLYMYOSITIS

Dermatomyositis and polymyositis are rare in pregnancy. After the onset of these diseases, fertility may be reduced and miscarriage more common. Flares may require drug treatment, but are not themselves associated with fetal loss. Dermatomyositis is a subacute systemic weakness of the proximal limb and trunk muscles associated with skin lesions (**9.11, 9.12**). In established dermatomyositis or polymyositis, an increase in rash activity and/or proximal muscle weakness may occur in 50% of affected patients in pregnancy, while remission may occur in another 20% in pregnancy[2]. There may be increased subcutaneous calcification in polymyositis during pregnancy (**9.13, 9.14**). Dermatomyositis may also occur for the first time during pregnancy[2].

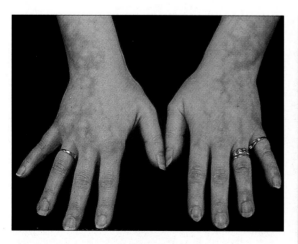

9.9 Livedo reticularis. This is a cutaneous hallmark of antiphospholipid antibodies. As well as miscarriage and thrombosis, these antibodies may be associated with cardiac murmurs due to valvular vegetations.

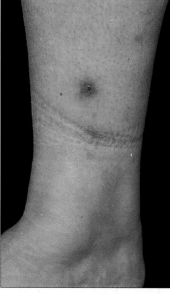

9.10 Cutaneous ulcers. Cutaneous ulcers, especially on the lower legs, which are notoriously persistent, are a less usual manifestation of antiphospholipid syndrome.

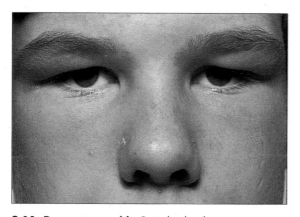

9.11 Dermatomyositis. Periorbital violescent (heliotrope) rash with associated edema.

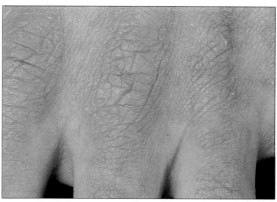

9.12 Gottron's papules. Erythematous purple papules on the dorsal aspects of the metacarpophalangeal and interphalangeal joints.

Fetal risk

Fetal loss due to miscarriage, stillbirth, or neonatal death (prematurity) occurs in over half of all cases[3]. Ishii *et al.*, however, suggest that pre-existing dermatomyositis or polymyositis does not present a great risk during pregnancy to either the mother or fetus, and that fetal mortality is increased when onset or relapse occur during pregnancy[4]. A significant improvement can usually be expected in the puerperium[5].

TREATMENT

Ideally, pregnancy should be planned at a time of remission, and the patient should be monitored closely throughout the pregnancy for clinical and laboratory signs of disease exacerbation. Prednisone, administered in minimal effective doses, is the mainstay of treatment for dermatomyositis and polymyositis. A dosage of 40mg daily may be required initially (about

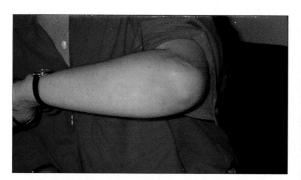

9.13 Polymyositis. Acceleration of subcutaneous calcification, shown here at the elbow, was noted by this young woman with polymyositis during pregnancy. The disease remained inactive in other respects.

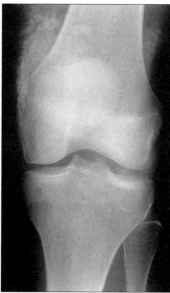

9.14 Polymyositis. Radiograph of knee of same patient as in **9.13**, showing calcification of subcutaneous tissues in lower thigh.

1mg/kg/day). Steroid treatment should be tapered cautiously (10% per month), particularly in the post-partum period, since an exacerbation may be precipitated by rapid withdrawal.

Although immunosuppressive agents (e.g. methotrexate, azathioprine and cyclophosphamide) are used as second-line treatments in the non-pregnant patient, they should be avoided during pregnancy (*see above*). After delivery, maintenance methotrexate should be considered for patients who require large doses of corticosteroids, and if the disease is severe or of long duration, a combination of steroid and immunosuppressive agent is now recommended.

EHLERS–DANLOS SYNDROME

Although Ehlers–Danlos syndrome and pseudoxanthoma elasticum are not regarded as 'connective tissue' tissues in the sense described above, they are included in this chapter for convenience. Ehlers–Danlos syndromes I–X are a group of inherited disorders of collagen metabolism, characterized by fragile skin and blood vessels, easy bruising, skin hyperelasticity, and joint hypermobility.

Women with Ehlers–Danlos types I (classic or gravis) and IV (ecchymotic or arterial) are particularly likely to develop complications during pregnancy such as postpartum bleeding, poor wound-healing, wound dehiscence, uterine lacerations, bladder and uterine prolapse, and abdominal hernias[6]. The rupture of major blood vessels, including the aorta and pulmonary artery, and rupture of the bowel or uterus can also occur, especially with type IV disease – in which maternal death can be as high as 25%[7]. A favourable outcome for pregnancy has been reported for type II (mitis) and type X (fibronectin abnormality) and possibly mild forms of the disease[6]. Avoidance of pregnancy has been recommended for women with types I and IV disease[8]. It is therefore important to categorize the patient's condition accurately so that the likely prognosis can be established.

The management of delivery for women with Ehlers–Danlos syndrome is difficult. Catastrophic complications are most likely to occur during labor, delivery, or in the first few days postpartum[7]. Although cesarean section is recommended for patients with types I and IV disease, it may not result in fewer complications than with vaginal delivery[7]. Early term-ination of pregnancy should be considered if ultrasound examination of the aortic root demonstrates more than 20% enlargement above the baseline, or a diameter greater than 4cm[8]. Zinc supplementation may be beneficial in some patients with type I disease[6].

PSEUDOXANTHOMA ELASTICUM

Pseudoxanthoma elasticum is a familial disease characterized by widespread degeneration of elastic tissue involving the skin (**9.15**), eye, gastrointestinal tract, and blood vessels. Case reports of pseudoxanthoma elasticum complicating pregnancy suggest that pregnancy may particularly aggravate the vascular effects of the disease[9]. The main complication during pregnancy is gastrointestinal bleeding with massive hematemesis[10]. Other complications include repeated epistaxis and congestive heart failure with ventricular arrhythmia.

There is no proven fetal risk in pseudoxanthoma elasticum, though intrauterine growth retardation associated with placental abnormalities has been reported[6]. As the complications of pseudoxanthoma elasticum in pregnancy relate to the vascular system, careful control of blood pressure may help to reduce the risk of hemorrhage.

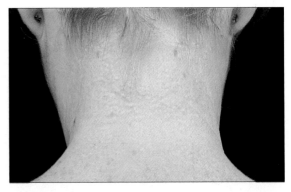

9.15 Pseudoxanthoma elasticum. The skin is loose and thickened like a plucked chicken. This is a rather subtle clinical change. The sides of the neck are characteristic sites.

REFERENCES

1 Hughes, G. R. V. The antiphospholipid syndrome: ten years on. *Lancet* 1993; **342**: 341–344.

2 Gutierrez, G., Dagnino, R., and Mintz, G. Polymyositis/dermatomyositis and pregnancy. *Arthritis Rheum.* 1984; **27**: 291–294.

3 Rosenzweig, B. A., Rotmensch, S., Binette, S. P., *et al.* Primary idiopathic polymyositis and dermatomyositis complicating pregnancy: diagnosis and management. *Obstet. Gynecol. Survey* 1989; **44(3)**: 162–170.

4 Ishii, N., Ono, H., Kawaguchi, T., *et al.* Dermatomyositis and pregnancy. Case report and review of the literature. *Dermatologica* 1991; **183**: 146–149.

5 Ohno, T., Imai, A., and Tamaya, T. Successful outcomes of pregnancy complicated with dermatomyositis. Case reports. *Gynecol. Obstet. Invest.* 1992; **33**: 187–189.

6 Winton, G. B. Skin diseases aggravated by pregnancy. *J. Am. Acad. Dermatol.* 1989; **20**: 1–13.

7 Rudd, N. L., Nimrod, C., Holbrook, K. A., *et al.* Pregnancy complications in type IV Ehlers-Danlos syndrome. *Lancet* 1983; i: 50–53.

8 Hammerschmidt, D. E., Arneson, M. A., Larson, S. L., *et al.* Maternal Ehlers-Danlos syndrome type X: successful management of pregnancy and parturition. *J.A.M.A.* 1982; **248**: 2487–248.

9 Berde, C., Willis, D. C., and Sandberg, E. C. Pregnancy in women with pseudoxanthoma elasticum. *Obstet. Gynecol. Survey* 1983; **38**: 339–344.

10 Lao, T. T., Walters, B. N. J., and de Swiet, M. Pseudoxanthoma elasticum and pregnancy: two case reports. *Br. J. Obstet. Gynaecol.* 1984; **91**: 1049–1050.

FURTHER READING

Buchanan, N. M. M., Khamashta, M., Kerslake, S., *et al.* Practical management of pregnancy in systemic lupus erythematosus. *Fetal Maternal Med. Review* 1993; **5**: 223–230.

Kean, W. F. and Buchanan, W. W. Pregnancy and rheumatoid disease. *Bailliere's Clinical Rheumatalogy* 1990; 4(1): 125–140.

Mitz, G. Dermatomyositis. *Rheum. Dis. Clin. N. Am.* 1989; **15**(2): 375–382.

Silman, A. J. Pregnancy and scleroderma. *Am. J. Reprod. Immunol.* 1992; **28**: 238–40.

ACKNOWLEDGEMENT

Figure **9.6** has been reproduced by kind permission of Dr. D. J. Atherton, The Hospital for Sick Children, London, UK.

10.
Vulvar Viral Disease in Pregnancy

Alison Taylor

MOTHER TO FETUS TRANSMISSION

Infections in pregnancy raise the specific question of transmission from the mother to the fetus. Transmission may occur *in utero*, perinatally or postnatally, by a variety of routes, including:

- Hematogenous spread across the placenta;
- Ascending infection from the lower genital tract;
- Following invasive investigative procedures, such as amniocentesis, chorionic villous sampling, or fetal blood sampling.

Although most of the components of the fetal immune system are present by the end of the first trimester, the fetal immune system is not fully developed. Fetal immunocompetence gradually increases with advancing gestation, but even at term, this is relatively reduced when compared with adults. Thus, infections that may be asymptomatic or have a benign clinical picture in the mother may have devastating effects in the fetus or neonate.

Antenatal viral infections can be associated with a risk of spontaneous abortion, congenital abnormalities, intrauterine growth retardation, intrauterine death, preterm delivery, or neonatal transmission. Different viral infections may be associated with specific clinical problems.

HERPES SIMPLEX VIRUS

CLINICAL FEATURES

The herpes simplex virus (HSV) is a double-stranded DNA virus which has two subtypes, HSV 1 and HSV 2. In common with other herpesviruses, such as varicella-zoster, cytomegalovirus and the Epstein–Barr virus, they have the capacity to establish latency and therefore produce recurrent disease.

Although, classically, HSV 1 is associated with oral infections and HSV 2 with genital herpes, there is in fact considerable crossover, and the two HSV types produce indistinguishable clinical pictures in respective sites. Up to 50% of genital herpes infections are found to be caused by HSV 1. Primary genital infection is acquired sexually, and manifests itself after an incubation period of 2–12 days.

The virus causes intraepithelial bullae to form, resulting in vesicles which may quickly rupture to form multiple small shallow ulcers (**10.1**). These vesicular or ulcerated lesions are surrounded by an area of erythema and inflammation, and can be extremely painful. They may be found on the external genitalia, buttocks, or cervix, and less commonly on the vaginal epithelium, or in the rectum as proctitis. Vulvitis may be associated with dysuria, which can be severe enough to inhibit micturition and cause urinary retention. The ulcers may become secondarily infected by bacteria. Viremic symptoms, such as general malaise and pyrexia, are more commonly, though not exclusively, seen with primary rather than recurrent infections. There is also more likely to be local lymphadenopathy.

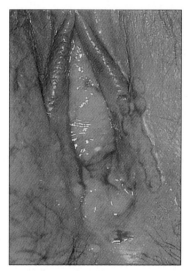

10.1 Herpes genitalis. Typical pattern of herpes genitalis erupting on the labium. The blister roofs have been lost, leaving typical 'punched-out' shallow lesions with a scalloped border.

RECURRENT EPISODES

After crusting over, the lesions usually resolve spontaneously within 10–21 days. The virus ascends the sensory neurons to the sacral ganglia, where it remains as a latent infection. Following reactivation of the infection and initiation of viral replication, the virus then travels back down the axons to the genital area to cause recurrent symptoms.

The mechanisms for viral reactivation are poorly understood, but recurrences are more likely to follow primary genital infection with HSV 2 rather than with HSV 1[1]. Eighty per cent of patients with a primary genital infection due to HSV 2 will have at least one recurrence[2]. In contrast, the rate of recurrence of HSV 1 infection on the genitalia is lower.

Although epidemiologic evidence has shown that 80% of the adult population have had primary gingivostomatitis, which is usually due to HSV 1, only about 20% will have a recurrent infection[3]. The risk of recurrent herpes labialis may be linked to human leukocyte antigen (HLA) status[4].

Recurrent episodes of infection may be triggered by stimuli such as exposure to ultraviolet light, local trauma, fatigue and stress, concurrent illness, and menstruation. In other cases, there are no obvious precipitating factors. Clinically, the lesions of secondary infections are the same as those of a primary attack, though they are generally less severe symptomatically and tend to resolve more quickly, within 5–10 days.

The pattern of recurrence is enormously variable; it can range from a single secondary attack to 6–12 episodes a year in a few patients. In general, recurrences tend to decrease in severity and frequency, with increasing time after the primary infection. In some patients, reactivation is subclinical, and the virus is shed asymptomatically[5-7]. There is also increasing evidence that other patients acquire HSV 2, without any overt history of a primary attack[8-11]. Patients with genital herpes can find recurrent attacks distressing and may develop long-term psychologic problems, particularly with sexual relationships[12].

DIAGNOSIS

Genital herpes is usually diagnosed by clinical inspection, and diagnosis may be confirmed by the viral culture of swabs taken from the lesions. Cultures are examined daily for evidence of a cytopathic effect and prolonged culture may be needed. The use of fluorescein isothiocyanate (FITC) conjugated monoclonal antibodies to HSV can speed up the detection and reporting rate[13]. Serologic tests are not usually helpful in adults, due to the high prevalence of HSV antibodies in the community. However, detection of HSV-specific IgM antibodies in neonatal serum may be the only early way of establishing whether or not perinatal transmission has occurred.

MATERNAL INFECTION

In general, the clinical picture of genital HSV infection is thought to be unaltered during pregnancy[13]. However, there have been sporadic reports of systemic HSV infection in pregnancy, such as encephalitis[14,15] or hepatitis[16,17]. These rare, but serious, complications of HSV infection are usually seen only in immunocompromised patients.

Other infections that are usually mild, but may be life-threatening during pregnancy, include influenza, varicella, hepatitis (A, B, and non-A, non-B), listeriosis, tuberculosis, and malaria. The fact that these are all intracellular infections suggests that subtle changes in cell-mediated immunity may occur in pregnancy[18,19], predisposing antenatal patients to severe infections normally seen in the elderly or immunocompromised. Although the duration of HSV recurrences does not change in pregnancy, there is some evidence that the frequency of recurrences increases with advancing gestation[6].

FETAL AND NEONATAL INFECTION

The management of a pregnant patient with a history of genital HSV is controversial. The risk of vertical transmission of a potentially fatal infection to the fetus has to be weighed against the risk to the mother of obstetric intervention, such as cesarean section.

Infection *in utero*

Rarely, maternal viremia results in maternofetal transmission by hematogenous transplacental spread, leading to congenital HSV infection. The sequelae can be spontaneous abortion, fetal malformations, intrauterine growth retardation, and perinatal death. Case reports have also suggested that congenital HSV infection can be acquired via ascending infection from the lower genital tract via intact membranes in babies delivered by cesarean section[20,21]. This assumption was based on histologic examination of the placenta and membranes which showed positive viral staining of cells in the subamniotic connective tissue, amniotic epithelium, and umbilical cord[20].

Neonatal HSV infection acquired *in utero* usually presents within the first 48 hours of life, while infection acquired during delivery generally presents clinically about 5–10 days later. The frequency of intrauterine infection has been estimated at about 5% of all babies with neonatal infection[22].

Perinatal Infection

Neonatal HSV infection occurs at a frequency between 1 in 500 and 1 in 10,000 births[23-27]. The incidence is generally higher in the USA than in Europe. Neonatal disease manifests itself as one of three forms[27]:

- Localized to the skin, eyes, and mouth;
- with CNS involvement (encephalitis);
- As disseminated disease, involving the liver, lungs, kidneys, gastrointestinal tract, pancreas, adrenal glands, and the heart, as well as widespread CNS involvement.

If untreated, disseminated disease carries the worst prognosis with a high mortality rate (50–70%), and a high morbidity in those who survive[28,29]. Early recognition of infections beginning in the skin or mucous membranes is essential, because 75% of cases will progress to disseminated disease if untreated[30]. In one series of 43 infants with neonatal HSV infection, only 12 (28%) had mothers with an antenatal history of genital herpes, and eight (19%) were delivered by cesarean section[31]. A high index of suspicion is therefore required, even when there are no previous risk factors.

Primary maternal HSV infection is more likely to result in transmission of virus to the neonate than in a recurrent or secondary episode. Studies have estimated a 50% risk of maternofetal transmission from a primary infection[32], and between 3 and 8% for recurrent disease[7,33,34]. Neonatal HSV infections acquired during a primary maternal infection are more likely to disseminate, and therefore have a poorer prognosis[33]. However, the risk of this is relatively low, as demonstrated by a prospective study which examined the incidence of primary maternal HSV 2 infections acquired during pregnancy[35]. The study found that four of 1580 women (0.25%) seroconverted during their pregnancy, three of them asymptomatically.

Some protection of the fetus and neonate is likely to be provided by maternal neutralizing antibodies in secondary maternal infections[7]. The maternal serum titer of HSV antibody has been shown to be predictive of a minimal level of antibody titer in cord blood at delivery[36], and may therefore help identify those infants at risk of serious infection. Neonatal HSV infection can be diagnosed by isolating the virus from skin lesions, cerebrospinal fluid, feces, urine, or nasopharyngeal secretions. Serologic tests for the presence of HSV-specific IgM antibodies may aid diagnosis in neonates who are initially asymptomatic, or who have been started on prophylactic antiviral therapy.

MANAGEMENT IN PREGNANCY

Screening

Until recently, screening during pregnancy was advocated for women with a history of genital HSV infection[37,38], and a program of weekly cervical swab cultures during the last five weeks of pregnancy was recommended by the Committee on Infectious Diseases for the American Academy of Pediatrics (1988).

However, the value of screening has been questioned[39,40]. These recommendations have now been withdrawn as a result of studies that showed screening is ineffective at predicting which patients with latent HSV infection will actively secrete virus at delivery[9,41,42]. It has been estimated that a national screening program in the USA would prevent only 1.8 cases of neonatal herpes annually, at a cost of more than $37 million per case prevented[43].

Since, at the current time, it is not possible to diagnose *in utero*-acquired infection before delivery, obstetricians and pediatricians need to maintain a high index of clinical suspicion, perinatally and postnatally, especially where a primary maternal infection has occurred during pregnancy.

Mode of Delivery

Currently, the best predictor of active virus shedding at the time of delivery appears to be the presence of clinical lesions within the lower genital tract. All patients should be carefully examined on admission to the delivery suite, and if any suspicious lesions are seen, swabs for HSV detection should be taken. Swabs should also be taken from women describing prodromal symptoms. Lesions on the buttocks can be associated with cervical shedding of the virus and should be included in this protocol[44].

Viral detection can be performed rapidly using electron microscopy, but if this is not possible or the result is not available at the time of delivery, patients with clinically suspicious lesions should be assumed to be excreting the virus. The current consensus of opinion is that these patients, and those with a positive swab, should deliver by cesarean section, unless the membranes have already been ruptured for more than four hours, after which time the protective effect of abdominal delivery will have been lost. All other patients with a history of genital HSV infection can receive vaginal delivery[5,45-47].

There is some evidence to suggest that fetal scalp electrodes are associated with an increased risk of neonatal HSV infection in this situation, and should be avoided if possible[7]. There has also been concern about the safety of regional anesthetic techniques, such as epidural or spinal block, for patients with active HSV infection at delivery. However, recent reports suggest that there is no increased risk of introducing HSV into the central nervous system with these techniques. These methods can be safely used for patients with active infection at the time of delivery[48,49].

Antiviral Therapy

Acyclovir is an antiviral agent with specific action against herpesviruses. It is a nucleoside that is rapidly phosphorylated by virus-specific thymidine kinase, after gaining access to an HSV-infected cell[50]. The phosphorylated acyclovir inhibits HSV-specific DNA polymerase, preventing further viral replication. Due to its highly specific, virus-dependent mode of activation, phosphorylated acyclovir is not found in uninfected cells. Therapy is therefore both effective and has few side effects.

Acyclovir can be administered topically, orally, or intravenously, although the topical form is only effective in primary infection. Oral acyclovir is most effective if used during the prodromal phase, which is usually missed by the time patients present with their first infection. It should be administered intravenously to immuno-compromised patients, 5 to 10mg/kg 8 hourly, to prevent dissemination.

Acyclovir can also be used for recurrent herpes infections. Episodic treatment is started by the patient as soon as she becomes aware of the prodromal symptoms, and can avert an attack or reduce the severity of the symptoms. Administration of the oral tablets, 200mg five times daily, can be used for these purposes. For patients who suffer frequent recurrences, continuous suppressive oral therapy with 400mg twice daily may be used for 6–12 months at a time.

Acyclovir has been used to treat severe complications of HSV infection in pregnancy, such as disseminated infection[51] and hepatitis[17]. There has also been interest in using acyclovir to suppress recurrences of HSV during pregnancy. Acyclovir apparently becomes concentrated in the amniotic fluid, without accumulation in the fetus, and no toxicity is seen in mothers or infants[52]. However, oral acyclovir administered after 37 weeks' gestation may fail to suppress asymptomatic shedding of HSV and transmission to the neonate[53]. One of the concerns about the use of prophylactic acyclovir in late pregnancy is that it may reduce the number of overt clinical attacks, without altering the incidence of asymptomatic shedding[50]. Further evaluation of acyclovir in pregnancy is needed.

HUMAN PAPILLOMAVIRUS

MATERNAL INFECTION

Despite the fact that genital warts are the most common vulvar viral condition, remarkably little has been written about human papillomavirus (HPV) infection in pregnancy. Anecdotally, genital warts are said to grow more rapidly in pregnancy and can become florid or hemorrhagic[54]. This could be related to a change in cellular immunity during pregnancy[19]. Very occasionally, warts may grow large enough to obstruct the birth canal, with the consequence that delivery has to be performed by cesarean section[55,56]. There is no known association between HPV infection and spontaneous abortion, intrauterine growth retardation, preterm delivery, or perinatal death.

The characteristic appearance of genital warts is shown in **10.2**. The lesions themselves may be present as small, irregular protrusions or may coalesce into thicker, rough-surfaced, 'warty' plaques of irregularly surfaced lesions (**10.3**). The verrucous surface is made up of a grossly hyperplastic epithe-

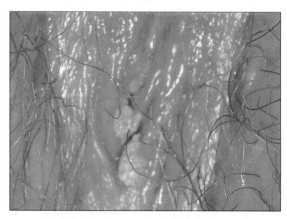

10.2 Genital warts. Two small condylomata acuminata are seen with their typical outline and roughened surface.

Vulvar Viral Disease in Pregnancy

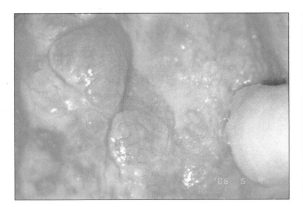

10.3 Genital warts. A small plaque of raised, HPV-infected epithelium on the labium. A colposcopic examination would demonstrate changes in the vascular pattern, which include 'open mosiac and acetowhite patterns'. The irregular surface contour is also visible.

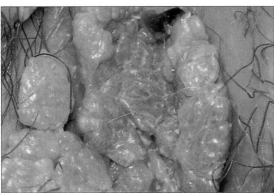

10.4 Genital warts. A collection of prominent condolymata acuminata are seen surrounding the introitus. Florid condylomata of this type are typical of those seen in pregnancy.

lium, which may be mistaken by the unwary as being precancerous (**10.4**). The lesion not only affects vulvar skin, but also commonly extends around the anus. It is not unusual to see the first attack of this complication develop during the first pregnancy.

There are conflicting reports as to whether there is an increased prevalence of genital HPV infection in pregnancy[57–60]. However, clinically apparent infections seem to occur more often during pregnancy and regress rapidly after delivery[61]. Hormonal effects may be important, as well as possible immunosuppression, as long-term users of oral contraceptives show an increased risk of developing HPV-related neoplasia[62].

Oncogenic Potential

The interest in HPV has increased in recent years because of its oncogenic potential[63]. For example, epidermodysplasia verruciformis is a rare, genetically determined, autosomal–recessive condition, with depressed cellular immunity and multiple cutaneous warts. Thirty-five per cent of affected patients will develop squamous cell carcinoma[64]. Human papillomavirus has been detected in the Buschke–Löwenstein tumor (*see also Chapter 20*), a low-grade, well-differentiated, slow-growing, squamous cell carcinoma of the genitalia or perianal area[65]. There is also a large body of circumstantial evidence linking HPV infection (particularly types 16, 18, 31, and 33) with an increas-

ed risk of cervical intraepithelial neoplasia (CIN) and cervical carcinoma, though a causal relationship has still to be established[66–69]. It is not yet known whether an increased prevalence of HPV infection and viral replication in pregnancy will increase the risk of CIN or cervical carcinoma. It is also difficult to gauge the clinical significance of the detection of HPV-DNA by sensitive methods, such as the polymerase chain reaction, in asymptomatic individuals[69].

FETAL AND NEONATAL INFECTION

Far less is known about the transmission of HPV to the fetus or neonate than of HSV. However, an association has been described between the presence of maternal genital warts and juvenile laryngeal papillomata[70-74]. Although rare, juvenile laryngeal papillomata cause significant morbidity and, occasionally, mortality in infected infants. HPV-DNA sequences have also been detected in the foreskins of clinically normal male neonates. This suggests that asymptomatic transmission of the virus may be more common than previously recognized[75]. Vertical transmission of HPV has been documented in a prospective study[76]. However, more long-term longitudinal studies are needed to establish the real risks of HPV infection to both pregnant women and their children.

MANAGEMENT IN PREGNANCY

HPV infection is very common and the presence of HPV-DNA in cells may not equate to a risk of clinical pathology. In the light of the above evidence, however, it seems prudent to treat genital warts whenever they are diagnosed, in order to minimize the reservoir of infection. There are many methods of treating genital warts, with variable efficacy. A major problem is the recurrence of warts after treatment.

Topical Treatment

One of the most commonly used methods of treating genital warts, podophyllin therapy, should be avoided at all stages of pregnancy. Administration during the first trimester has been associated with possible teratogenicity, and fetal death has been reported following its use in late pregnancy[77–79]. Trichloroacetic acid therapy (90%) is an alternative topical method which can be used safely in pregnancy. The keratolytic must be applied carefully because of the risk of ulceration and scarring. Pain on application is common.

Cryotherapy

Cryotherapy can be effective, does not require any anesthetic, and causes little or no scarring. It has been suggested as the first choice of therapy, as it has a higher cure rate than topical chemotherapy, and significantly fewer applications are required[80].

Surgical Methods

Surgical methods such as electrocautery, excision, and laser, are performed under local or general anesthetic, but bleeding may be an increased risk in pregnancy. Colposcopically guided laser ablation has the advantages of greater precision over the site and depth of treatment, rapid healing, and minimal scarring. It has been advocated as the method of choice for treating genital warts in pregnancy[56], and high success rates of up to 97%, with recurrence rates as low as 3%, have been reported[81]. There is not enough evidence available to justify cesarean section delivery in pregnant women with HPV infection.

MOLLUSCUM CONTAGIOSUM

This viral condition is extremely common and is often found in children. It is spread by direct contact and can be sexually transmitted. It can occur anywhere on the body, but sexually acquired disease may be found in the genital area. The lesions are small, pearly, umbilicated papules, which may be mistaken for genital warts (**10.5**). The disease is benign and self-limiting once an antibody response is mounted, and treatment may not be required. On the other hand, lesions in immunosuppressed patients (e.g. with AIDS) may be florid and extensive.

There is no evidence to suggest that there are any adverse effects associated with infection during pregnancy. However, presumably, if genital lesions are present, they could infect the infant through contact during delivery. If treatment is required, cryotherapy or inoculation with phenol, cantharidin or iodine can be used.

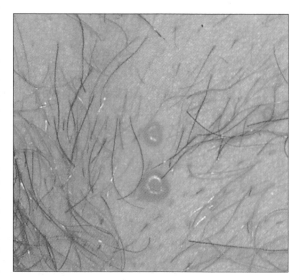

10.5 Molluscum contagiosum.

REFERENCES

1 Reeves, W. C., Corey, L., Adams, H. G., *et al.* Risk of recurrence after first episode of genital herpes. Relation to HSV type and antibody response. *N. Engl. J. Med.* 1981; **305**: 315–319.

2 Russell, J. The management of recurrent genital herpes. *Br. J. Sexual Med.* 1992; **19**: 147–150.

3 Lamey, P. J. Herpes labialis. *Br. J. Sexual Med.* 1993; **20**: 24–26.

4 Galina, G., Cumbo, V., Messina, P., *et al.* MHC-linked genetic factors (HLA-B35) influencing recurrent circumoral herpetic lesions. *Dis. Markers* 1987; **5**: 191–197.

5 Catalano, P. M., Merritt, R. N., and Mead, P. B. Incidence of genital herpes simplex virus at the time of delivery in women with known risk factors. *Am. J. Obstet. Gynecol.* 1991; **164**: 1303–1306.

6 Harger, J. H., Amortegui, A. J., Meyer, M. P., *et al.* Characteristics of recurrent genital herpes simplex infections in pregnant women. *Obstet. Gynecol.* 1989; **73**: 367–372.

7 Brown, Z. A., Benedetti, J., Ashley, R., *et al.* Neonatal herpes simplex virus infection in relation to asymptomatic maternal infection at the time of labor. *N. Engl. J. Med.* 1991; **324**: 1247–1252.

8 Cunningham, A. L., Lee, F. K., Ho, D. W., *et al.* Herpes simplex virus type 2 antibody in patients attending antenatal or STD clinics. *Med. J. Aust.* 1993; **158**: 525–528.

9 Garland, S. M. Neonatal herpes simplex: Royal Women's Hospital 10-year experience with management guidelines for herpes in pregnancy. *Aust. NZ. J. Obstet. Gynecol.* 1992; **32**: 331–334.

10 Frenkel, L. M., Garratty, E. M., Shen, J. P., *et al.* Clinical reactivation of herpes simplex virus type 2 infection in seropositive pregnant women with no history of genital herpes. *Ann. Internal Med.* 1993; **118**: 414–418.

11 Kulhanjian, J. A., Soroush, V., Au, D. S., *et al.* Identification of women at unsuspected risk of primary infection with herpes simplex virus type 2 during pregnancy. *N. Engl. J. Med.* 1992; **326**: 916–920.

12 Goldmeier, D., Johnson, A., Byrne, M., *et al.* Psychosocial implications of recurrent genital herpes simplex virus infection. *Genitour. Med.* 1988; **64**: 327– 330.

13 Carrington, D. Viral infections in pregnancy. In: MacLean, A. B. (ed.) *Clinical Infection in Obstetrics and Gynaecology.* Oxford: Blackwell Scientific Publications, 1990; p.39–71.

14 Frieden, F. J., Ordorica, S. A., Goodgold, A. L., *et al.* Successful pregnancy with isolated herpes simplex virus encephalitis: case report and review of the literature. *Obstet. Gynecol.* 1990; **75**: 511–513.

15 Roman-Campos, G., Navarro de Roman, L. I., Toro, G., *et al.* Herpes encephalitis in pregnancy. *Am. J. Obstet. Gynecol.* 1979; **135**: 158–159.

16 Jacques, S. M. and Qureshi, F. Herpes simplex virus hepatitis in pregnancy: a clinicopathologic study of three cases. *Human Pathol.* 1992; **23**: 183–187.

17 Klein, N. A., Mabie, W. C., Shaver, D. C, *et al.* Herpes simplex virus hepatitis in pregnancy. Two patients successfully treated with acyclovir. *Gastroenterology* 1991; **100**: 239–244.

18 MacLean, A. B. Infection and the antenatal patient. In: MacLean, A. B. (ed.) *Clinical Infection in Obstetrics and Gynaecology.* Oxford: Blackwell Scientific Publications, 1990, p21–38.

19 Purtilo, P. T., Hallgren, H. M., and Yunis, E. J. Depressed maternal lymphocyte response to phytohaemagglutinin in human pregnancy. *Lancet* 1972; **i**: 769–771.

20 Hyde, S. R. and Giacoia, G. P. Congenital herpes infection: placental and umbilical cord findings. *Obstet. Gynecol.* 1993; **81**: 852–855.

21 Stone, K. M., Brooks, C. A., Guinan, M. E., *et al.* National surveillance for neonatal herpes simplex virus infections. *Sex. Trans. Dis.* 1989; **16**: 152–156.

22 Baldwin, S. and Whitley, R. J. Intrauterine herpes simplex virus infection. *Teratology* 1989; **39**: 1–10.

23 Whitley, R. J. Neonatal herpes simplex virus infection. *J. Reprod. Med.* 1986; **31**: 426–432.

24 Yeager, A. S., Arvin, A. M., Urbani, L. J., *et al.* Relationship of antibody to outcome in neonatal herpes simplex virus infections. *Infect. Immun.* 1980; **29**: 532–538.

25 Sullivan-Bolyai, J., Hull, H. F., Wilson, C., *et al.* Neonatal herpes simplex virus infection in King County, Washington: increasing incidence and epidemiologic correlates. *J. Am. Med. Assoc.* 1983; **250**: 3059–3062.

26 Arvin, A. M., Yeager, A. S., and Bruhn, F. W. Neonatal herpes simplex infection in the absence of mucocutaneous lesions. *J. Pediatr.* 1982; **100**: 715–721.

27 Whitley, R. J. Neonatal herpes simplex virus infections: pathogenesis and therapy. *Pathol. Biol. (Paris)* 1992; **40**: 729–734.

28 Sutton, A. and Turner, T. Neonatal infection. In: MacLean, A. B. (ed.) *Clinical Infection in Obstetrics and Gynaecology.* Oxford; Blackwell Scientific Publications, 1990; p173–194.

29 Whitley, R. J., Nahmias, A. J., Visintine, A. M., *et al.* The natural history of herpes simplex virus infection of mother and newborn. *Pediatrics* 1980; **66**: 489–494.

30 Arvin, A. M. Antiviral treatment of herpes simplex infection in neonates and pregnant women. *J. Am. Acad. Dermatol.* 1988; **18**: 200–203.

31 Koskiniemi, M., Happonen, J. M., Jarvenpaa, A. L., *et al.* Neonatal herpes simplex virus infection: a report of 43 patients. *Pediatr. Infect. Dis. J.* 1989; **8**: 30–35.

32 Nahmias, A. J., Josey, W. E., Naib, Z. M., *et al.* Perinatal risk associated with maternal genital herpes simplex virus infection. *Am. J. Obstet. Gynecol.* 1971; **110**: 825–827.

33 Arvin, A. M. Relationships between maternal immunity to herpes simplex virus and the risk of neonatal herpesvirus infection. *Rev. Infect. Dis.* 1991; **13**: 953–956.

34 Prober, C. G., Sullender, W. M., Yasukawa, L. L., *et al.* Low risk of herpes simplex virus infections in neonates exposed to the virus at the time of vaginal delivery. *N. Engl. J. Med.* 1987; **318**: 887–891.

35 Boucher, F. D., Yasukawa, L. L., Bronzan, R. N., *et al.* A prospective evaluation of primary genital herpes simplex virus type 2 infections acquired during pregnancy. *Pediatr. Infect. Dis. J.* 1990; **9**: 499–504.

36 Harger, J. H., Guevarra, L., and Armstrong, J. A. Neutralizing antibody to herpes simplex in pregnant women and their neonates. *J. Perinatol.* 1990; **10**: 16–19.

37 Woolley, P. D., Lacey, H. B., and Helsen, K. Screening pregnant women for genital herpes. *Int. J. Sex. Trans. Dis. AIDS* 1992; **2**: 287–288.

38 Woolley, P. D, Bowman, C. A, Hicks, D. A., *et al.* Virological screening for herpes simplex virus during pregnancy. *Br. Med. J.* 1988; **296**: 1642–1643.

39 Carney, O. and Mindel, A. Screening pregnant women for genital herpes. *Br. Med. J.* 1988; **296**: 1643.

40 Kelly, J. Genital herpes during pregnancy. *Br. Med. J.* 1988; **297**: 1146–1147.

41 Arvin, A. M., Hensleigh, P. A., Prober, C. G., *et al.* Failure of antepartum maternal cultures to predict the infant's risk of exposure to herpes simplex at delivery. *N. Engl. J. Med.* 1986; **315**: 796–800.

42 Prober, C. G., Sullender, W. M., Yasukawa, L. L., *et al.* Use of routine viral cultures at delivery to identify infants exposed to herpes simplex infection. *N. Engl. J. Med.* 1988; **318**: 887–891.

43 Binkin, N. J. and Koplan, J. P. The high cost and low efficacy of weekly viral cultures for pregnant women with recurrent genital herpes: a reappraisal. *Med. Decision Making* 1989; **9**: 225–230.

44 Suarez, M., Briones, H., and Saaevdra, T. Buttock herpes. High risk in pregnancy. *J. Reprod. Med.* 1991; **36**: 367–368.

45 Randolph, A. G., Washington, A. E., and Prober, C. G. Cesarean delivery for women presenting with genital herpes lesions: efficacy, risks and costs. *J. Am. Med. Assoc.* 1993; **270**: 77–82.

46 Jeffries, D. J. Intrauterine and neonatal herpes simplex virus infection. *Scand. J. Infect. Dis.* 1991; **80**(suppl.): 21–26.

47 Sperling, R. S. and Berkowitz, R. L. Obstetric management of women with a history of recurrent genital herpes. *Am. J. Perinatol.* 1989; **6**: 275–277.

48 Bader, A. M., Camann, W. R., and Datta, S. Anesthesia for cesarean delivery in patients with herpes simplex virus type-2 infections. *Regional Anesthesiol.* 1990; **15**: 261–263.

49 Crosby, E. T., Halpern, S. H., and Rolbin, S. H. Epidural anesthesia for cesarean section in patients with active recurrent genital herpes simplex infections: a retrospective review. *Can. J. Anes.* 1989; **36**: 701–704.

50 Brown, Z. A. and Baker, D. A. Acyclovir therapy during pregnancy. *Obstet. Gynecol.* 1989; **73**: 526–531.

51 Grover, L., Kane, J., Kravitz, J. et al Systemic acyclovir in pregnancy: a case report. *Am. J. Obstet. Gynecol.* 1985; **65**: 284–287.

52 Frenkel, L. M., Brown, Z. A., Bryson, Y., *et al.* Phamacokinetics of acyclovir in the term human pregnancy and neonate. *Am. J. Obstet. Gynecol.* 1991; **164**: 569–576.

53 Haddad, J., Langer, B., Astruc, D., *et al.* Oral acyclovir and recurrent genital herpes during late pregnancy. *Obstet. Gynecol.* 1993; **82**: 102–104.

54 Roberts, J. Genitourinary medicine and the obstetrician and gynaecologist. In: MacLean, A. B. (ed.) *Clinical Infections in Obstetrics and Gynaecology.* Oxford; Blackwell Scientific Publications, 1990: p.237–254.

55 Wilson, J. Extensive vulvar condylomata acuminata necessitating cesarean section. *Aust. NZ. J. Obstet. Gynecol.* 1973; **13**: 121–124.

56 Osborne, N. G. and Adelson, M. D. Herpes simplex and human papillomavirus genital infections: controversy over obstetric management. *Clin. Obstet. Gynecol.* 1990; **33**: 801–811.

57 Schneider, A., Hotz, M., and Gissmann, L. Increased prevalence of human papillomaviruses in the lower genital tract of pregnant women. *Intnal. J. Cancer* 1987; **40**: 198–201.

58 Rando, R. F., Lindheim, S., Hasty, L., *et al.* Increased frequency of detection of human papillomavirus deoxyribonucleic acid in exfoliated cervical cells during pregnancy. *Am. J. Obstet. Gynecol.* 1989; **161**: 50–55.

59 Peng, T. C., Searle, C. P., Shah, K. V., *et al.* Prevalence of human papillomavirus infections in term pregnancy. *Am. J. Perinatol.* 1990; **7**: 189–192.

60 Kemp, E. A., Hakenewerth, A. M., Laurent, S. L., *et al.* Human papillomavirus prevalence in pregnancy. *Obstet. Gynecol.* 1992; **79**: 649–656.

61 Gary, R. and Jones, R. Relationship between cervical condylomata, pregnancy and subclinical papillomavirus infection. *J. Reprod. Health* 1985; **30**: 393–399.

62 WHO. Invasive cervical cancer. *Br. Med. J.* 1985; **290**: 961–965.

63 Lynch, P. The oncogentic potential of human papillomavirus. *Am. J. Dermatopathol.* 1982; **4**: 55–60.

64 Lutzner M.A. Epidermolysis verricuformis. *Bull. Cancer* 1978; **65**: 169–182.

65 Boxer, R.J. and Skinner, D.G. Condylomata acuminita and squamous cell carcinoma. *Urology* 1977; **9**: 72–78

66 Zur Hausen, H. Human genital cancer : Synergism between two virus imfections or synergism between a virus infection and an initiating event. *Lancet* 1982; **i**: 1370–1372.

67 Francheschi, S., Doll, R., Gallwey, J., *et al.* Genital warts and cervical neoplasia: an epidemiological study. *Br. J. Cancer* 1983; **48**: 621–628.

68 Bauer, H. M., Ting, Y., and Greer, C. E. Genital human papillomavirus infection in female university students as determined by a PCR based method. *J. Am. Med. Assoc.* 1991; **265**: 472–477.

69 Reeves, W. C., Brinton, L. A., and Garcia, M. Human papillomavirus infection and cervical cancer in Latin America. *N. Engl. J. Med.* 1989; **320**: 1437–1441.

70 Kaufman, R.S., and Balogh, K. Verrucae and juvenile laryngeal papillomas. *Archives of Otolaryngology* 1969; **89**: 90–91.

71 Cook, T.A., Cohn, A.M., and Brunschwig, J.P. Laryngeal papilloma: Etiologic and therapeutic considerations. *Annals of Otolaryngology* 1973; **82**: 649–655

72 Quick, C.A., Krzyzek, R.A., Watts, S.L., and Faras, A.J. Relationship between condylomates and laryngeal papillomata. *Annals of Otolaryngology* 1980; **89**: 467–471.

73 Cohn, A.M., Kos J.T., Taber, L.H. and Adam, E. Recurring laryngeal papilloma. *American Journal of Otolaryngology* 1981; **2**: 129–132.

74 Mounts, P. and Shak, K. V. Respiratory papillomatosis: etiological relation to genital tract papillomavirus. *Prog. Med. Virol.* 1984; **29**: 90.

75 Roman, A. and Fife, K. Human papillomavirus DNA associated with foreskins of normal newborns. *J. Infect. Dis.* 1986; **153**: 855–861.

76 Pakarian, F., Kaye, J., Cason, J., *et al.* Cancer associated human papillomaviruses: perinatal transmission and persistence. *Br. J. Obstet. Gynecol.* 1994; **101**: 514–517.

77 Chamberlain, M.J., Reynolds, A.L., and Teoman, W.B., Toxic effects of podophyllum application in pregnancy. *British Medical Journal* 1972; **3**: 391–392.

78 Bargman, H. Is podophyllin a safe drug to use and can it be used during pregnancy? *Arch. Dermatol.* 1988; **124**:1718.

79 Karol, M.D.,Connor, C.S.,Watanabe, A.S., and Murphrey, K. Podophyllum: suspected teratogenicity from topical application. *Clinical Toxicology* 1980; **16**: 283–286.

80 Bashi, S. A. Cryotherapy versus podophyllin in the treatment of genital warts. *Intnal. J. Dermatol.* 1985; **24**: 535–536.

81 Bellina, J. H. The use of carbon dioxide laser in the management of condylomata acuminata with eight year follow up. *Am. J. Obstet. Gynecol.* 1983; **147**: 375–378.

ACKNOWLEDGEMENT

Figures **10.1** and **10.5** are reproduced from S.A. Morse, A.A. Moreland & S.E. Thompson *Atlas of Sexually Transmitted Diseases* (Figs 2.12a and 12.41b), Gower, New York 1990.

11.
Vulvar Anatomy

Michael Katesmark & Peter Braude

INTRODUCTION

The vulva comprises the structures that form the female external genitalia, namely:
- The mons pubis;
- The labia majora and minora;
- The clitoris;
- The vestibule;
- The Bartholin's (greater vestibular) glands (**11.1**).

It lies centrally within the anterior perineal triangle. This is the region defined by the symphysis pubis anteriorly, the pubic rami laterally, and the transverse perineal muscles posteriorly. A sling of fibers derived from the levator ani muscle sweeps behind the vagina to form the sphincter vaginae, with the remaining space laterally filled by the urogenital diaphragm.

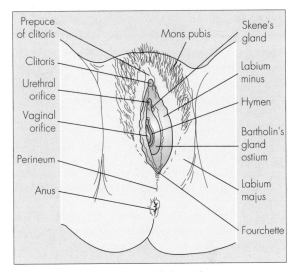

11.1 Schematic diagram of the vulva.

LABIA MAJORA

The labia majora correspond to the scrotum in the male, and form two thick folds of skin lateral to the vaginal orifice. Anteriorly, they fuse to form the mons pubis overlying the pubic bone; posteriorly, they blend into the perineal skin. The lateral aspects contain numerous hair follicles and apocrine sweat glands, with sebaceous glands lying predominantly within the medial walls.

LABIA MINORA

The labia minora are two vascular, rugose slips of skin, which lie just within the labia majora. The lateral portions of the inner minora contain tiny sebaceous glands, which may be perceived as small yellowish papules when the skin is stretched. Devoid of hair follicles and adipose tissue, the labia minora are hyperpigmented in the adult and may vary considerably in size (**11.2**).

Anteriorly, they fuse around the clitoris, forming the prepuce above it and the frenulum below. Poster-

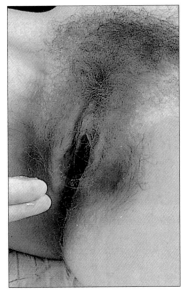

11.2 Normal vulva.

iorly, they form a lip of skin known as the fourchette. At birth, under the influence of maternal estrogens, the female genitalia are prominent and occasionally pigmented. Throughout infancy, the labia majora and mons pubis gradually lose their generous layer of adipose tissue and remain devoid of hair.

CLITORIS

This sensitive and erectile organ is the homolog of the male penis. With the exception of a urethra, it contains all the structures found in the penis, with the following less developed and thus less easily demonstrated, namely:

- The spongy, vascular corpora cavernosa (originating from the inferior pubic rami), which form most of the body;
- The vestigial ischiocavernosus and bulbospongiosus muscles, which insert into the body and root, respectively.

Densely supplied by cutaneous branches of the pudendal nerve, the clitoris becomes engorged and highly sensitive during intercourse.

VESTIBULE

Parting of the labia reveals the oval orifice known as the vestibule (**11.3**), into which opens the urethra anteriorly, the ducts of Skene's glands lateral to the urethra, the ducts of Bartholin's glands posterolaterally, and the vagina. At the posterior fourchette, tiny finger-like projections (papillae) may often be seen. Sweeping around the vestibule on each side, rudimentary fibers of the bulbospongiosus muscles envelop a rich plexus of veins and loose areolar tissue called the bulb of the vestibule (**11.4**), which be-

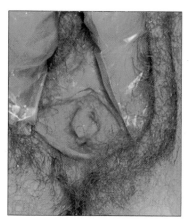

11.3 Separation of the labia minora reveals the vestibule.

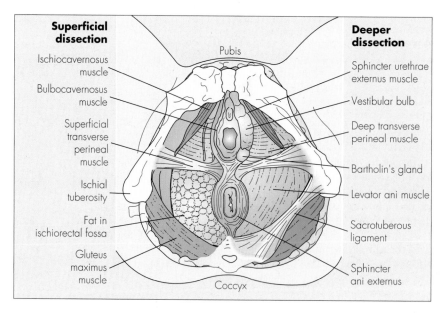

11.4 Dissection of the perineum shows the superficial muscles, the position of Bartholin's gland and the vestibular bulb.

Superficial dissection

Ischiocavernosus muscle
Bulbocavernosus muscle
Superficial transverse perineal muscle
Ischial tuberosity
Fat in ischiorectal fossa
Gluteus maximus muscle

Pubis
Coccyx

Deeper dissection

Sphincter urethrae externus muscle
Vestibular bulb
Deep transverse perineal muscle
Bartholin's gland
Levator ani muscle
Sacrotuberous ligament
Sphincter ani externus

comes engorged during sexual arousal and may become varicose during pregnancy.

At the posterior base of each bulb, about two-thirds of the way down the lateral wall, lie the mucus-secreting Bartholin's glands. Normally impalpable, their 2cm ducts may easily become blocked in adulthood resulting in dramatic swelling and infection (*see Chapter 20*).

PERINEAL BODY

The fibromuscular perineal body, formed from the common insertion of the superficial muscles of the perineal pouch, both supports the lower part of the vagina and divides it from the anal canal. The perineal body is often the subject of trauma at delivery, either due to tearing or to episiotomy, and afterwards the fourchette may be left deficient (**11.5**)

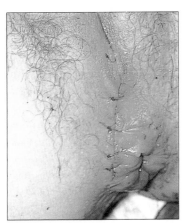

11.5 Repair of episiotomy following low forceps delivery.

EMBRYOLOGY OF THE LOWER GENITAL TRACT

Until five weeks' gestation, the urogenital and alimentary systems share a common reservoir, the cloaca. This is derived from the caudal region of the hindgut (**11.6**), and is separated from the surface by the cloacal membrane. Between five and seven weeks' gestation, mesoderm migrates distally to become the urogenital septum, dividing the cloaca into the larger

urogenital sinus and the anorectal canal. The septum eventually fuses with the cloacal membrane to produce the anal membrane and the urogenital membrane, with the genital tubercle superiorly (**11.7**). The close embryologic derivation of the vulva and anus is reflected in the common blood supply and nerve supply of these areas, and the numerous dermatologic conditions that afflict both organs in a similar manner.

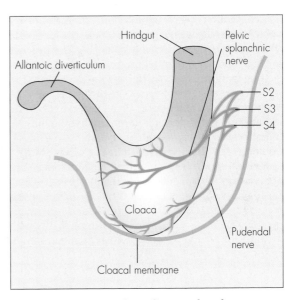

11.6 The cloaca at about five weeks of intrauterine life.

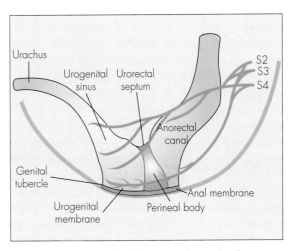

11.7 The cloaca after the seventh week of intrauterine life.

The mesonephric ducts (wolffian ducts) open into the cloaca on about the 26th day of gestation. This subdivides the urogenital sinus into a cranial portion continuous with the allantois (the vesicourethral canal), which subsequently forms the bladder and part of the urethra, and a caudal portion, the urogenital sinus 'proper', which gives rise to the lower one-third of the vagina. Two solid outgrowths of the sinus – the sinovaginal bulbs – elongate as the fetus grows, eventually meeting the lower tip of the fused paramesonephric (müllerian) ducts to form a solid epithelial column that represents the future vagina.

Canalization of the vagina occurs relatively late (at approximately 26 weeks' gestation), with the formation of lacunae that progressively coalesce. The process is occasionally incomplete, resulting in vaginal septae, or more rarely, partial or total occlusion. The hymen is thought to represent the region between the urogenital sinus and the canalized derivatives of the sinovaginal bulbs. In rare cases, the hymen may be imperforate, causing the retention of menstrual blood behind it and giving rise to a hematocolpos (**11.8**).

The external genitalia of the male and female are structurally indistinguishable (the indifferent stage) until about 12 weeks of gestation. By about seven weeks, the cloacal membrane is divided into a urogenital membrane and an anal membrane (**11.9**), with an anterior genital tubercle, two symmetric genital

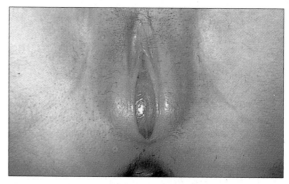

11.8 Imperforate hymen resulting in the accumulation of menstrual blood.

folds and two genital swellings. The secondary sex characteristics appear earlier in the male than in the female fetus, probably reflecting the earlier functional activity in the testis. The Y-chromosome induces the gonad to become a testis in the genetically male fetus. The differentiation of the external genitalia in the female occurs because of the absence of this positive male-determining effect. Exposure to exogenous or endogenous androgens at this critical stage will result in a variable degree of masculinization (**11.10**).

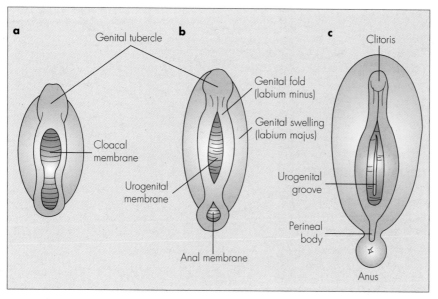

11.9 Stages in the development of external genitalia in the female: (a) at five weeks; **(b)** at seven weeks; **(c)** at 12 weeks.

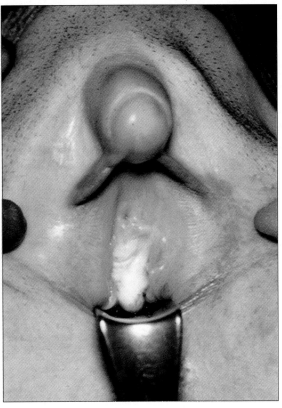

11.10 An enlarged clitoris as a result of virilization.

BLOOD SUPPLY

The arterial supply to the vulva is derived largely from the internal pudendal artery, a terminal branch of the internal iliac artery. Entering the buttock beneath the gluteus maximus muscle, it arches round the ischial spine, passes through the lesser sciatic notch, and approaches the perineum in the roof of the ischiorectal fossa, lying in company with the pudendal nerve in the pudendal (Alcock's) canal (**11.11**). The named terminal branches, from posterior to anterior, are:

- The inferior rectal artery, passing medially from the pudendal canal to supply the anal canal and sphincter;
- The perineal and transverse perineal branches, passing anteromedially over the ischiorectal fossa, and piercing the superficial perineal muscles to supply the anal and vaginal sphincters, anterior fibers of the levator ani muscle, and the skin of the perineal body and posterior labia;
- The artery of the bulb, passing through the urogenital diaphragm to the bulb of the vestibule;
- Two terminal branches, the dorsal and deep arteries, to the clitoris.

There is also a supply from the superficial and deep external pudendal arteries, which arise from the femoral artery. The pudendal artery and its branches are

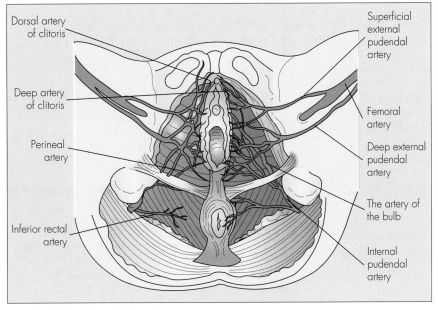

11.11 Blood supply of the vulva.

Dorsal artery of clitoris

Deep artery of clitoris

Perineal artery

Inferior rectal artery

Superficial external pudendal artery

Femoral artery

Deep external pudendal artery

The artery of the bulb

Internal pudendal artery

accompanied by a rich network of veins, ultimately draining into the internal iliac veins. This, together with the extensive anastomoses to the peripheral branches of the inferior gluteal and external pudendal arteries, ensures a plentiful blood supply and accounts for the rapid healing of the vulva following trauma, such as childbirth.

NERVE SUPPLY

The nerve supply to the vulva and perineum arises mainly from the anterior rami of the five sacral and coccygeal nerves, with a small input from the fifth lumbar nerve via the ilioinguinal nerve. The vulva itself is supplied by branches of the pudendal nerve, formed from the second, third and fourth sacral nerve roots, and representing the largest component of the anterior sacrococcygeal plexus. Lying just medial to the pudendal artery, the nerve follows an almost identical path through the pudendal canal to reach the vulva (**11.12**). Recognized branches are:

*   The inferior rectal nerve, supplying the external anal sphincter and the perianal skin;
*   The perineal nerve, divided into a superficial branch (supplying the skin over the perineal body) and a larger deep branch, supplying the levator ani muscle, the external sphincters, the vaginal muscles, and ultimately the erectile tissue of the bulb;
*   The dorsal nerve to the clitoris, running close to the pubic arch to enter the root of the clitoris.

All the nerves communicate extensively and there is considerable overlap with the ilioinguinal nerve anteriorly, the posterior cutaneous nerve of the thigh centrally, and the anococcygeal nerve posteriorly.

A knowledge of the course through the pudendal canal is important in producing a pudendal block using local anesthetic agents. Access can be gained through the skin lateral to the perineal body, or through the lateral wall of the vagina, using a specially guarded pudendal needle (**11.13**).

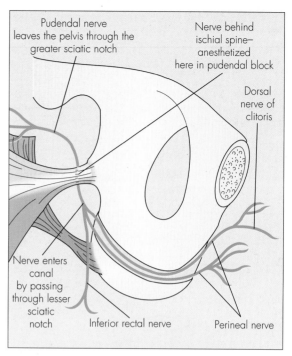

11.12 The course of the pudendal nerve.

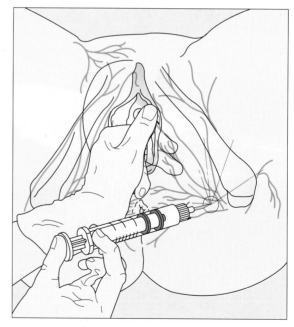

11.13 Site of injection for pudendal nerve block.
Practically, the needle would be inserted through the vaginal wall and not through the skin as shown, which is simply done for clarity.

LYMPHATIC DRAINAGE

The vulva, in common with the lower trunk and back, the buttock, the perineum, and the anus (below the mucocutaneous junction), drains via superficial lymphatic channels to the superficial inguinal (groin) nodes. These lie just distal to the inguinal ligament on each side. From here, drainage occurs through the saphenous opening in the fascia lata femoris to the deep inguinal (femoral) nodes that lie in the femoral triangle (**11.14**).

A constant feature is the medially placed Cloquet's node, guarding the entrance to the femoral canal. Lymph channels then pass beneath the inguinal ligament to reach the external iliac nodes, and subsequently the common iliac nodes, and thence the para-aortic nodes. Drainage from the labia occurs predominantly to the ipsilateral inguinal nodes, whereas midline structures, the fourchette and particularly the clitoris, may drain bilaterally.

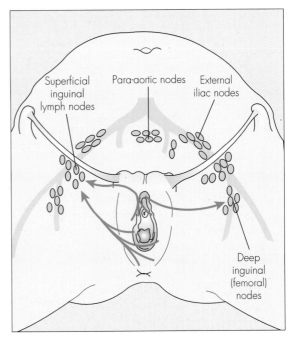

11.14 Schematic diagram of the lymphatics of the vulva. Extensive intercommunication exists between the lymphatics of each side.

ACKNOWLEDGEMENTS
Figures **11.2**, **11.5** and **11.8** are reproduced from E.M. Symonds and M.B.A. Macpherson *Color Atlas of Obstetrics and Gynaecology* (Figs 1.25, 7.48 and 10.1), Mosby–Wolfe, London 1994.
Figures **11.3** and **11.10** are reproduced from V.R. Tindall *Colour Atlas of Clinical Gynaecology* (Figs 6 and 27), Wolfe, London 1981.

12.
Classification of Cutaneous Vulvar Disorders – International Society for the Study of Vulvovaginal Disease (ISSVD)

C. Marjorie Ridley

HISTORY

The need for a coherent, logical yet simple classification for vulvar disease is self-evident; without it, comparison of data is impossible, fruitful discussion impeded, and practical management of the patient made difficult. Towards the end of the 19th century, vulvar diseases began to be described. A profusion of terms arose, devised by gynecologists and dermatologists – but without mutual knowledge, let alone agreement. In the mid-20th century attempts were made to formulate a working classification. The history of how this situation arose and how it has been resolved – at least to some extent – is described in detail elsewhere[1].

EVOLUTION OF EARLY SCHEMES

Briefly, the main problems of classification were:
- To clarify the entity of lichen sclerosus;
- To recognize lichen simplex and lichenification; these are both thickening of the skin in response to itching and rubbing, the former being a primary condition, and the latter a secondary condition, superimposed on an itchy dermatosis;
- To declare redundant many of the terms used up until then.

The outcome was the scheme described originally by Gardner and Kaufman, and formalized as that of The International Society for the Study of Vulvovaginal Disease (ISSVD)[2]. The ISSVD is a multidisciplinary and international body, which had come into being in 1970 (as the International Society for the Study of Vulvar Disease) with the development of a rational classification as one of its aims.

In retrospect, the original classification (**Table 12.1**) had two drawbacks. It was essentially histopathologic and omitted consideration of many known cutaneous disorders, the diagnosis of which was of obvious clinical and academic importance. For example, lichen simplex and lichenification were concealed under 'hyperplastic dystrophy'. Moreover, with its categories of 'atypia', it came to be seen as overlapping the territory of neoplastic disease. This trespass was emphasized by the development of interest in vulvar intraepithelial neoplasia (VIN), as a result of its increased frequency and increased recognition in the last 20 years.

CLASSIFICATION OF VULVAR INTRAEPITHELIAL NEOPLASIA

In turn, efforts were made to create a satisfactory classification of VIN, and to ensure that such a classification was not drawn into the maelstrom of conflicting views on the role of the human papillomavirus in VIN. The result, jointly agreed by the ISSVD and the International Society of Gynecologic Pathologists (ISGYP), is set out in **Table 12.2**[3]. The grades of VIN 1, 2 and 3 correspond to what had previously been referred to as mild and moderate atypia (VIN 1 and 2), and severe atypia and carcinoma *in situ* (VIN 3). Vulvar intraepithelial neoplasia was defined as follows:
- 'VIN is characterized by loss of epithelial cell maturation with associated nuclear hyperchromasis, pleomorphism, cellular crowding and ab-

---

1 Hyperplastic dystrophy
    (a) Without atypia
    (b) With atypia
2 Lichen sclerosus
3 Mixed dystrophy (lichen sclerosus with foci of epithelial hyperplasia)
    (a) Without atypia
    (b) With atypia
*A detailed histologic definition and description were given for each of the conditions noted above. Atypia was classified as mild, moderate, or severe, and with or without dystrophy.

This classification is no longer recommended[2].

Table 12.1 ISSVD Classification of Vulvar Dystrophies 1976[2].

Category	Description
VIN 1	Mild dysplasia
VIN 2	Moderate dysplasia
VIN 3	Severe dysplasia, carcinoma *in situ*

Table 12.2 Classification of VIN 1986[3].

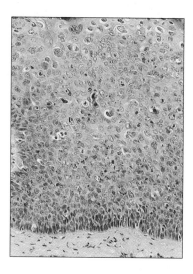

12.1 VIN 3. Full-thickness changes.

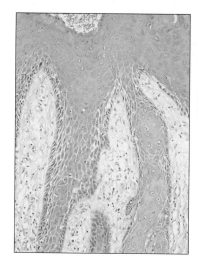

12.2 VIN 3. Differentiated type. Note the changes are confined to the basal and parabasal area, with keratin pearls in the rete ridges.

normal mitosis. Dyskeratotic cells, 'corps ronds', hyperkeratosis and parakeratosis may be present.' The subdivisions of VIN were further defined:

- VIN 1. Nuclear hyperchromasia is present, with cellular disarray involving the lower one-third of the epithelium; mitoses within the lower one-third of the epithelium are often seen and are usually abnormal.
- VIN 2. Nuclear hyperchromasia is present, with cellular disarray involving up to the lower two-thirds of the epithelium; mitoses within the lower two-thirds of the epithelium are often seen and are usually abnormal.
- VIN 3. Nuclear hyperchromasia is present, with cellular disarray involving more than the lower two-thirds of the epithelium; mitoses within the area of cellular disarray are often seen and are usually abnormal; the term carcinoma *in situ* is usually reserved for cases that have near-full or full-thickness epithelial changes (**12.1**).

Further comments elaborated on these definitions:

'The term differentiated type (i.e. VIN 3, severe dysplasia, differentiated type) is recommended for those cases that have cells with prominent eosinophilic cytoplasm, often with keratin or 'pearl-like' changes within the involved epithelium. These changes are usually seen near the tips of the rete ridges in the lower third of the epithelium (**12.2**). The epithelial cell nuclei in these areas usually have prominent nucleoli with vesicular, rather than coarsely clumped, chromatin. The more superficial epithelium may show some maturation. It is recommended that cases with such findings be classified as VIN 3.

Although the terms Bowen's disease, erythroplasia of Queyrat, and carcinoma simplex are included under the general heading of VIN, they are not preferred terms. The term Bowenoid papulosis, though controversial, is not accepted as a pathologic term; however, it is recognized that the term, as used by some dermatologists, refers to cases of VIN associated with multiple papule formation. Use of the terms Bowenoid papulosis or Bowenoid dysplasia is not recommended by the Society (*ISSVD*) for either clinical or pathologic use. The association of condyloma acuminatum should not influence the diagnosis or grading of VIN. When koilocytotic change or condyloma acuminatum occurs adjacent to or within a VIN lesion, it is recommended that a statement to that effect be made and that such terms as condylomatous dysplasia not be used.'

This classification will probably be modified in time. The criteria for the diagnosis of types 1 and 2 are somewhat arbitrary and these grades are probably of no great clinical significance; there is a danger that the existence of these terms may result in inappropriate treatment. There is some evidence[4] that a solitary patch of VIN in an older patient is of more clinical significance in terms of progression to malignancy than are the multiple, often HPV-related patches in younger patients, and this judgement cannot be reflected in the purely descriptive terminology described. Also, no attention is paid to the condition of the surrounding skin – whether normal or showing HPV infection or lichen sclerosus. It may be that the differentiated type of VIN 3 has especial significance as a forerunner of malignancy in lichen sclerosus[4].

EXTRAMAMMARY PAGET'S DISEASE AND MELANOMA *IN SITU* (NON-SQUAMOUS VIN)

The classification of VIN also includes extramammary Paget's disease (**12.3**) and melanoma *in situ*, i.e. non-squamous VIN. Although often difficult to diagnose clinically and histologically, the inclusion of these conditions in the classification is uncontroversial.

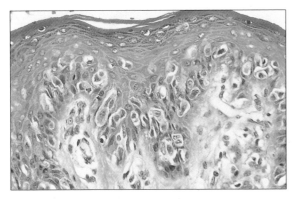

12.3 Extramammary Paget's disease.

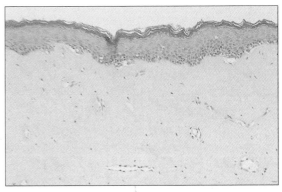

12.4 Lichen sclerosus.

SUPERFICIALLY INVASIVE SQUAMOUS CELL CARCINOMA OF THE VULVA (STAGE 1A)

Finally, the category of superficially invasive squamous carcinoma of the vulva should be noted briefly. This is defined as a single lesion measuring 2cm or less in diameter and with a depth of invasion of 1mm or less. The depth of invasion is measured:'... as the distance from the epithelial stromal junction of the adjacent, most superficial dermal papillae to the deepest point of invasion of tumor'.

The term 'thickness of tumor' is defined as '... the measurement from the surface of the tumor, or granular layer when a keratin layer is present, to the deepest point of invasion. The measurement of the diameter of the tumor should include invasive tumor only and not adjacent VIN.' The term 'microinvasive' is imprecise and should not be used. The importance of a Stage 1A tumor, as defined above, is that lymphatic metastasis is not part of the definition of the lesion, and therefore treatment by wide local excision should be effective and safe.

SQUAMOUS CELL CARCINOMA OF THE VULVA

Classification of squamous cell carcinoma is not relevant to this account of cutaneous lesions, and is currently under discussion between the ISSVD and the International Federation of Obstetricians and Gynecologists (FIGO). However, it is hoped that future developments in the classification of neoplastic lesions will pay attention to underlying vulvar conditions, and will help the clinician in selecting therapies that are more individualized and less uncompromisingly radical than at present.

CURRENT CLASSIFICATION OF NON-NEOPLASTIC CONDITIONS

The discussion now returns to the latest developments in the classification of non-neoplastic disease, following its separation from VIN. Although the concept of vulvodynia and its subdivisions, notably vestibulitis[5], has been developed, the objective and physical status of the disease are uncertain, and so it is not considered here under the heading of cutaneous disorders. Vulvodynia is discussed in *Chapter 14*.

Discussion between the ISSVD and ISGYP has resulted in the agreed following classification for the non-neoplastic conditions (**Table 12.3**)[6]. Additional comments on this new scheme are made in the form of footnotes to the main text, as follows:

'Mixed epithelial disorders may occur. In such cases, it is recommended that both conditions be reported. For example, lichen sclerosus (**12.4**) with associated squamous cell hyperplasia (formerly classified as mixed dystrophy) should be reported as lichen sclerosus with squamous cell hyperplasia. Squamous cell hyperplasia with associated VIN (formerly hyperplastic dystrophy with atypia) should be diagnosed as VIN ... Squamous cell hyperplasia is used for those instances in which hyperplasia is not attributable to a more specific tissue process. Specific lesions or dermatoses involving the vulva (e.g. psoriasis,

---

1 Lichen sclerosus (lichen sclerosus et atrophicus)
2 Squamous cell hyperplasia (formerly hyperplastic dystrophy)
3 Other dermatoses

Table 12.3 Classification of Non-Neoplastic Epithelial Disorders of Skin and Mucosa 1989[6].

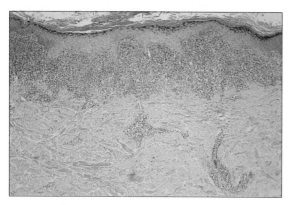

12.5 Lichen planus.

lichen planus (**12.5**), lichen simplex chronicus, *Candida* infection, condyloma acuminatum) may include squamous cell hyperplasia, but should be diagnosed specifically and excluded from this category because of their pathognomonic characteristics.'

This scheme too may be improved in the course of time. In general, dermatologists would like to see the category of squamous cell hyperplasia abolished in the conviction that all vulvar lesions can and should be described exactly – as are their counterparts on other areas of the body. Clearly, not all pathologic findings would be neatly diagnostic, but simple descriptive reports would be sufficient for doubtful cases. Until a formal revision is agreed upon, however, the classification should be adhered to as it stands, since vulvar disease cannot properly be studied without consistency and uniformity in reporting it.

REFERENCES

1 Ridley, C. M. General dermatological conditions and dermatoses of the vulva. In: Ridley, C. M. (ed.) *The Vulva*. Edinburgh: Churchill Livingstone, 1988, p.188–193.
2 Friedrich, E. G. New nomenclature for vulvar disease. *Obstet. Gynecol.* 1976; **47**: 122–124.
3 Wilkinson, E. J., Kneale, B., and Lynch, P. J. Report of the ISSVD terminology committee. *J. Reprod. Med.* 1986; **31**: 973–974.
4 Leibowitch, M., Neill, S., Pelisse, M., *et al.* The epithelial changes associated with squamous cell carcinoma of the vulva: a review of the clinical, histological and viral findings in 78 women. *Br. J. Obstet. Gynaecol.* 1990; **97**: 135–139.
5 McKay, M., Frankman, O., Horowitz, B. J., *et al.* Vulvar vestibulitis and vestibular papillomatosis; report of the ISSVD committee on vulvodynia. *J. Reprod. Med.* 1991; **36**: 413–415.
6 Ridley, C. M., Frankman, O., Jones, I. S. C., *et al.* New nomenclature for vulvar disease: report of the committee on terminology. *Am. J. Obstet. Gynecol.* 1989; **160**: 769.

ACKNOWLEDGEMENT

Figure **12.2** has been reproduced by kind permission of Dr C. H. Buckley, and Figures **12.1** and **12.3–12.5** by kind permission of Dr P. H. McKee.

13.
Vulvar Manifestation of Skin Disorders (Non-Neoplastic Epithelial Disorders)

Marilynne McKay

This group of disorders includes conditions that are familiar to dermatologists trained to seek diagnostic clues elsewhere on the skin. With practice, the non-dermatologist can recognize and treat these diseases with greater ease. **Table 13.1** summarizes the differential diagnosis of the vulvar disorders discussed in this chapter, and also outlines treatment.

PSORIASIS

Psoriasis (**13.1–13.3**) is usually easy to recognize, but lesions will look different on various parts of the body. Red plaques have silvery scales on dry skin, such as the elbows and knees, but appear gray-white and macerated in intertriginous areas. In these areas, fissures and cracks often cause discomfort. Involvement of the gluteal cleft is common in psoriasis, and lesions may also occur on knees, elbows, and the scalp. Nail pitting may be a diagnostic clue, even when skin involvement is minimal. *Psoriatic arthritis* occurs in less than 15% of patients. It is similar to rheumatoid arthritis, but it is predominantly distal, involving the fingers and toes. Reiter's disease should be considered when arthritis, acropustulosis, and ankylosing spondylitis occur with psoriasiform genital lesions. *Pustular psoriasis* is an unusual type of psoriasis that looks very much like *Staphylococcus* or

Candida infection. Reiter's disease may also have a pustular component.

Treatment
For lesions on the extremities and trunk, topical therapy with a mid- to high-potency steroid preparation is the usual mainstay of treatment. Vulvar lesions usually respond well to mid-potent steroids (e.g. triamcinolone acetonide, 0.1%) and should be tapered

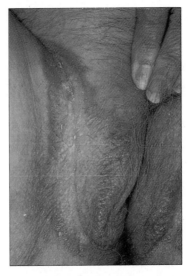

13.2 Intertriginous psoriasis. Thick scaly plaques in intertriginous folds with a sharply defined border are typical of psoriasis. These areas are easily traumatized and fissuring is common. Note: ungloved fingers in these photographs are the patient's own.

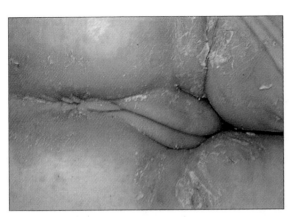

13.1 Intertriginous psoriasis. Extensive scaling and erythema of gluteal cleft and vulva. The patient should be examined carefully for other stigmata of psoriasis (plaques on the knees, elbows, scalp; nail pitting.)

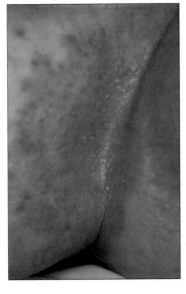

13.3 Pustular psoriasis of the vulva and inner thigh. This eruption may be indistinguishable from that of Reiter's disease, especially when there are symptoms of arthritis together with pustular lesions of the palms and soles. (These pustules were sterile and continued to erupt despite anticandidal treatment.)

Diagnosis	Onset	Symptoms	Appearance	Other areas affected	Treatment
Psoriasis	Chronic and recurrent	Painful if fissured	Thick, red scaly plaques with distinct margins	Scalp, knees, elbows, sacrun, nails	Topical steroids (triamcinolone 0.1%), systemic derm Rx if severe
Seborrheic dermatitis	Chronic and recurrent	Minimal	Thin reddish plaques with brannish scale	Scalp, central face, axillae	Dandruff shampoos, hydrocortisone 1% cream
Pityriasis versicolor	Chronic and recurrent	Minimal	Thin reddish plaques with furry scale	Trunk, shoulders; pigment variable	Topical imidazole creams twice daily until clear for one week
Intertrigo (chafing)	Acute	Tender	Erythema, sometimes petechiae	May follow clothing lines	Cool compress, bland emollient or hydrocortisone; avoid allergens
Intertrigo (chronic)	Chronic and recurrent; especially in obese	Moderate itching	Thin reddish plaques (erythrasma); if pruritic, may lichenify	Axillae	For erythrasma, topical or systemic erythromycin; mild soaps, talc, cortisone cream
Dermatitis (irritant or allergic contact)	Acute; may be recurrent	Itching	Microvesicular eruption which becomes dry and scaly; lasts 2–3 weeks	Other areas of contact	Cool compress, bland emollient or hydrocortisone; avoid allergens
Dermato-phyte (Tinea)	Acute or chronic	Itching, variable	Scaly plaques with inflammatory border	Usually spreads to adjacent areas	Topical imidazole creams twice daily until clear for one week; systemic griseofulvin if extensive
Candida vulvitis	Acute; may be recurrent in susceptible patients	Itching and burning	Bright erythema, swelling satellite pustules; vaginal discharge may be absent	Inflammatory area, sometimes axillae. Oral thrush	Topical imidazole creams for vulva and vagina for one week; systemic fluconazole if persistent
Lichen simplex chronicus	Chronic	Intense bouts of itching	Thick leathery plaques with enhanced skin markings, diffuse margins	May occur elsewhere if patient has a history of atopic dermatitis	Clobetasol 0.05% twice daily for one month then daily for one month, then 1–3 times weekly as needed; check often for vaginal *Candida*
Steroid-rebound dermatitis	Occurs after using steroids for several months	Burning	Pebbly, fine-textured erythema; accentuation of sebaceous glands	Similar lesions can occur on face if steroids have been applied there	Discontinue topical steroid – may need to taper by decreasing potency and/or frequency
Lichen planus	Chronic	Sometimes itchy, sore-ness at intoitus	Erosive mucosal surfaces; violescent papules or white reticulate pattern	Lacy white oral and vulvar mucosa. Papules common on wrists and shins	Biopsy for diagnosis; topical steroids; cream or suppositories
Lichen sclerosus	Chronic	May itch or burn; often asymptom-atic	White, wrinkly, atrophic, often petechial. Perianal 'keyhole' pattern	Usually none. Rarely generalized with confetti white spots on wrists, trunk, extremities	Clobetasol 0.05% twice daily for one month, then daily for one month, then 1–3 times weekly as needed
Paget's disease	Chronic and progressive	Minimal	Red, moist-appearing plaque with scaling	Local cutaneous spread; tumor cells may involve adjacent structures	Surgical excision; topical agents (e.g. 5-fluorouracil) are not curative

Table 13.1 Differential Diagnoses of Vulvar Dermatoses.

rapidly to hydrocortisone, 1% or 2.5%. Ultraviolet light therapy, while effective for the rest of the body, is difficult to administer to vulvar lesions. With severe involvement of the entire body, systemic therapy may be required (e.g. methotrexate, oral retinoids).

SEBORRHEIC DERMATITIS

Scaling and erythema are the most common manifestations of seborrhea, but immunosuppressed patients may have particularly exuberant lesions, with extensive red plaques and dry scaling (**13.4–13.7**). It is rare for seborrheic dermatitis to occur only on the geni-

talia. Other areas that should be examined include the eyebrows, nasolabial folds, and the periauricular and posterior hairline. Axillary involvement is common when genital lesions are present. A potassium hydroxide preparation of lesional scale may reveal the short hyphae and spores of tinea versicolor (*Pityrosporum ovale*, previously *Malassezia furfur*). This is probably a commensal organism that thrives in an environment rich in sebaceous oils.

Treatment

Topical treatment is usually effective. Mainstays of therapy are keratolytic agents ('dandruff' shampoos containing selenium sulfide, zinc pyrithione, or keto-

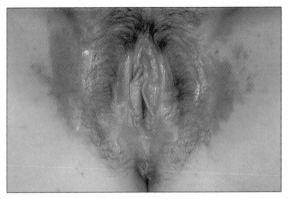

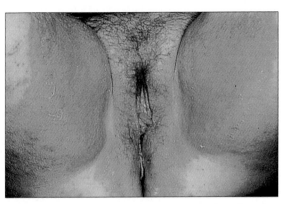

13.4 Seborrheic dermatitis, showing erythema of the vulva and intertriginous areas. This looks very much like psoriasis, but the typical scale is lacking. The patient also had lesions on the face and inframammary area, which were typical of seborrheic dermatitis. If there had also been scaling psoriatic plaques on the knees and elbows, this would have been called 'sebo-psoriasis'.

13.5 Exuberant seborrheic eczema on the vulva. This degree of involvement suggests secondary infection with *Candida* and/or immunosuppression.

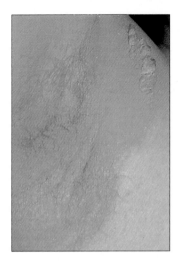

13.6 Axillary psoriasis. This would be indistinguishable from axillary seborrheic dermatitis, without the characteristic thick psoriatic scales at the edge of the lesion. The rest of the skin should be examined for typical lesions.

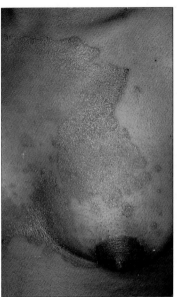

13.7 Extensive trunkal seborrheic dermatitis. There is post-inflammatory pigmentation in this postpartum patient, who developed this extensive eruption during the last trimester of her pregnancy. Although inframammary involvement is common, central chest lesions are uncommon in women. There was no evidence of *Pityrosporum ovale* in scale taken from the lesions.

conazole) and/or anti-inflammatory topical hydrocortisone preparations (hydrocortisone, 1% cream or lotion.)

PITYRIASIS (TINEA) VERSICOLOR

This common fungal infection (**13.8**) of the topmost layer of the skin (stratum corneum) recurs in susceptible individuals. There is some evidence that the responsible microorganism, *Pityrosporum ovale*, may preferentially grow where sebaceous gland output is highest. Superinfection with *P. ovale* might explain why seborrheic dermatitis is so exuberant in immunosuppressed patients, who are presumably less able to control the inflammatory response. It is unclear, however, whether the organisms are the cause of the increased seborrheic output, or are simply found in greater concentration where there is greater sebaceous gland production.

Treatment
Treatment with topical antifungals or keratolytic agents, such as sulfur and salicylic acid-containing soaps, is usually effective, but treatment must often be repeated monthly, especially in climates where temperature and humidity are high.

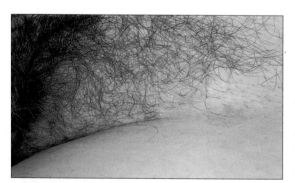

13.8 Tinea (pityriasis) versicolor of the vulva. The fine scale and salmon patches are very similar to seborrhea, but microscopic examination of lesional scale revealed *P. ovale*. There were no lesions on the trunk.

INTERTRIGO

This term refers to the skin changes that develop in intertriginous areas (**13.9,13.10**) because of chafing and chronic inflammation. Sometimes, there is also a fungal or bacterial infection, usually tinea, *Candida*, or *Corynebacterium minutissimum* (erythrasma).

Obese sedentary individuals and active athletes are both likely to have problems with intertrigo – the common factor is occlusion and rubbing together of skin surfaces. Ectomorphic bodybuilders with bulging muscles are more susceptible to intertrigo than are thin endomorphic runners.

Treatment
Keeping the area clean and dry, reducing friction with talcum powder, and treating secondary infection with the appropriate medication are all effective ways to control the problem.

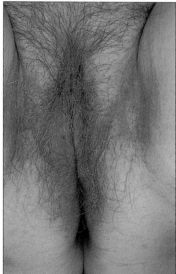

13.9 Intertrigo. The patient complained of irritation with heat and tight clothing. There was no evidence of *Candida* or tinea infection, and her condition improved with the use of talcum powder and loose cotton underwear.

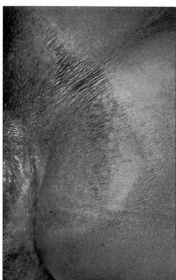

13.10 Chronic intertrigo. Postinflammatory hypopigmentation and hyperpigmentation of chronic intertrigo. Variations in pigmentation may be seen as inflammatory. Cutaneous conditions flare and resolve, especially in patients with darkly pigmented skin.

CONTACT DERMATITIS

There are two different types of contact dermatitis: allergic and irritant. Allergic contact dermatitis is due to a cell-mediated (type IV) allergic reaction – it takes 48–72 hours after the exposure to develop the rash. Only someone sensitized to a substance will develop allergic contact dermatitis, and the dermatitis will occur every time the patient encounters that substance (**13.11**).

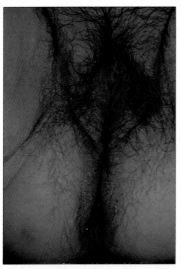

13.11 Chronic contact dermatitis to preservative (ethylenediamine) in topical cream.

An irritant reaction, on the other hand, only occurs if the skin's barrier function is compromised; it will happen to almost everyone under the same circumstances (like the stinging of vinegar on chapped hands). When the skin is intact, the irritant reaction is reduced or eliminated. The complaint of immediate stinging when something is applied to the skin is typical of an irritant reaction; although the skin may be sensitive, it does not mean the patient is truly allergic to that substance (i.e. will react every time it is encountered).

The cutaneous eruption of allergic contact dermatitis lasts for between two and three weeks. Outbreaks lasting only a few days are more likely to be eczema. If episodes seem continuous, patch testing may be necessary to discover the allergen.

STEROID REBOUND DERMATITIS

Characterized by intense erythema and the complaint of stinging or burning, this problem is the result of 'rebound' from high-potency topical steroids (**13.12–13.14**). These preparations cause local vasoconstriction. When the effect wears off, vessels relax and dilate with resulting erythema. Patients may interpret this as a worsening of their condition, and thus apply steroids more often than recommended.

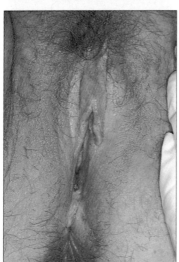

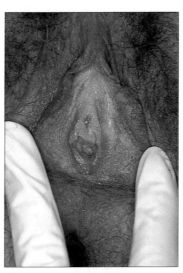

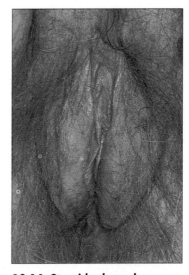

13.12 Steroid rebound dermatitis surrounding lichen sclerosus (LS) on the vulva. The patient had used 2% testosterone ointment daily for four years and complained of burning discomfort for the past six months. The LS was still active and the surrounding skin shows the fine-textured papular erythema typical of steroid rebound.

13.13 Steroid rebound dermatitis with burning of the inner labia minora after a high-potency topical steroid (fluocinonide, 0.05% cream) had been applied for two months to skin which was not lichenified and only mildly symptomatic.

13.14 Steroid rebound dermatitis with burning of the labia majora after a high-potency topical steroid (desoxymethasone, 0.25% cream) had been applied for three months for treatment of erosive vaginitis.

Almost all high- or 'super-potent' steroids will cause rebound dermatitis, but susceptible individuals (those with rosacea-like complexions) may develop steroid rebound from mid- or even low-potency preparations. Hydrocortisone, 1% or 2.5%, rarely causes problems with steroid rebound, even if used daily. Superinfection with *Candida* can also be a problem when using steroids, so if itching accompanies erythema, a vaginal culture should be considered (*see **Appendix B** for discussion of steroid potencies*).

DERMATOPHYTE (TINEA CRURIS)

Tinea infections (**13.15–13.17**) typically begin as inflammatory blisters or pustules which spread concentrically. The center of the lesion dries, becomes scaly, and heals, while the periphery continues to expand with small blisters or pustules. It may be difficult to find fungal hyphae at the active border because the inflammatory reaction is too great; lesional scale is best for identifying tinea.

Most patients have recurrences of tinea because they have not adequately treated the infection. Treatment typically takes about a month, which surprises many patients. It is good advice to recommend twice-daily treatment 'for at least a week after it looks like the rash has gone'. This will be more likely to eradicate hyphae that have penetrated hair follicles – a frequent source of reinfection.

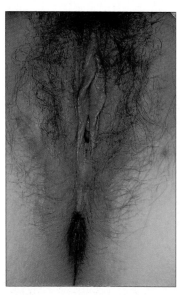

13.15 Annular margin of tinea on the vulva. Lesions of tinea are often subtle in women with normal immune systems. A high index of suspicion should be maintained and appropriate diagnostic tests should be done before treating lesions with topical steroids.

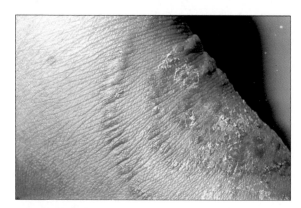

13.16 Annular tinea lesion. Vesicles and pustules at the advancing edge of a typical scaly plaque represent an inflammatory reaction, which subsequently subsides, leaving dry scales behind. Microscopic examination of the blister roof or dry scales may reveal fungal hyphae.

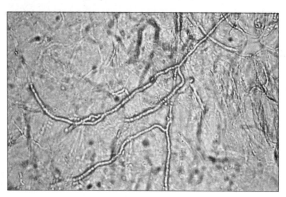

13.17 Dermatophyte (tinea cruris), showing a microscopic view of branched hyphae among cleared keratinocytes as they appear in a positive potassium hydroxide (KOH) preparation of lesional scale.

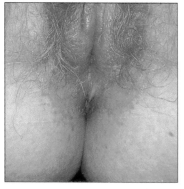

13.18 *Candida* vulvovaginitis. Intense erythema and edema around the introitus, perineum, and perianal areas. The discrete erythematous macules at the active borders are resolving pustules.

CANDIDA VULVOVAGINITIS

Candida vulvovaginitis (**13.18–13.20**) is very common and is usually associated with suppression of the normal cutaneous and gastrointestinal flora with antibiotic therapy. Immunosuppression is another factor, and diabetics are very likely to have problems with recurrent candidiasis (*see also* **18.3**). The typical eruption is a bright erythema with edema around the vagina and vulva. Pustules on an erythematous base are often dotted at the periphery of the primary plaque or erosive area. A Gram stain of a pustule will generally reveal budding yeast forms, confirming the diagnosis.

LICHEN SIMPLEX CHRONICUS

Lichen simplex chronicus (LSC) (**13.21**, **13.22**) is the most common of the vulvar dermatoses that contain the word 'lichen' in their name. This word is merely descriptive, and was originally used to evoke the botanical image of a rough-surfaced lichen heaped on a smooth-surfaced rock.

Each of the three skin diseases (lichen simplex chronicus; lichen sclerosus, LS; and lichen planus, LP) is histologically distinct. A dermatopathologist should have no difficulty in distinguishing between them, so it is reasonable to do a biopsy if the diag-

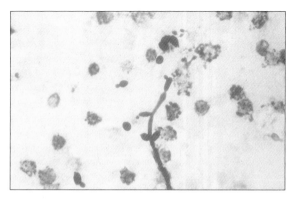

13.19 *Candida.* Periodic-acid Schiff (PAS) stain of budding yeast and pseudohyphae seen in *Candida albicans* vulvovaginitis.

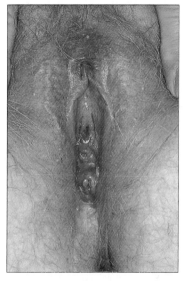

13.20 *Candida vulvovaginitis.* Low-grade erythema of the vulva with no evidence of vaginal discharge. The patient complained of postcoital irritation, with swelling and itching around the time of menses. She had asthma and often took oral corticosteroids. A KOH smear and vaginal culture revealed *C. albicans*.

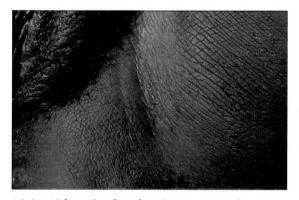

13.21 Lichen simplex chronicus (LSC). Leathery changes of intertriginous skin as a result of chronic rubbing and scratching. Note the accentuation of normal skin lines, one of the hallmarks of LSC.

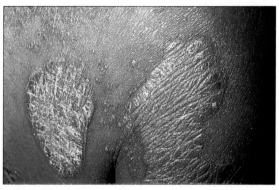

13.22 Psoriasis. Thick scaly plaques with increased skin markings. Unlike the plaques of LSC, psoriasis plaques are sharply demarcated and patients rarely complain of itching. (Bleeding can usually be induced by scratching or peeling scale from a psoriatic plaque. This is called Auspitz' sign, a diagnostic test for psoriasis.)

nosis is unclear. With a little practice, however, they are usually easy to distinguish from one another clinically. A pathology report noting 'hyperkeratosis and parakeratosis' usually refers to LSC. This non-specific description is of the cutaneous change seen when the patient has persistently rubbed or scratched the skin, producing the secondary change called lichenification. Clinically, the skin has a leathery appearance with accentuation of the normal skin markings.

LICHEN PLANUS

The classic description of lichen planus (LP) (**13.23–13.25**) is the 'five P's: Purple Polygonal Papules and Plaques that are Pruritic'. Lesions usually occur on the inner wrists and anterior shins. On the oral and vulvar mucosa, a lacy white pattern or erosions are typical, and some patients may have lesions limited to the mucosa (*see Chapter 17*).

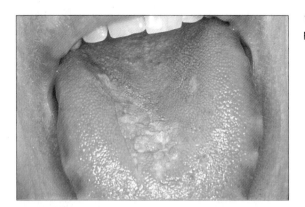

13.23 Oral lichen planus of the tongue. Whitish plaques are seen centrally.

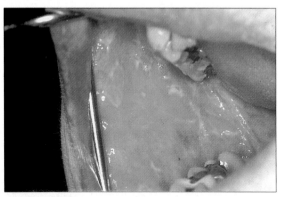

13.24 Oral lichen planus. Thin whitish linear streaks (Wickham's striae) are seen on the buccal mucosa. This is not usually symptomatic unless it is erosive.

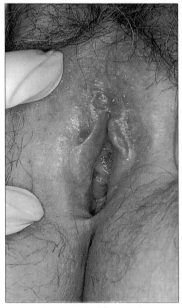

13.25 Vulvar lichen planus. Mucosal erosions of the vulvar vestibule and vagina are typical. Apparent loss of the posterior labia minora is due to adhesions developing after cutaneous erosion. This patient also had oral lesions of LP.

LICHEN SCLEROSUS

Lichen sclerosus (LS) (**13.26,13.27**) is one of the major vulvar dermatoses. The epidermis is atrophic, white and wrinkly, while the dermis is thickened and sclerotic. Typically, the disorder involves only the vulva and/or anus (keyhole pattern), but the trunk can also be involved with morphea-like white plaques. If a patient has had vulvar LS for many years, it is less likely that she will develop generalized LS (*see Chapter 16*).

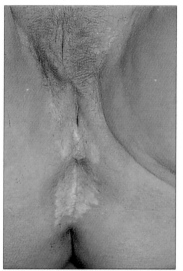

13.26 Lichen sclerosus. In this patient, there is well-circumscribed, white, atrophic change around the vulva and perianal skin. It can be distinguished from vitiligo because the latter is simply loss of pigment from normal skin, whereas LS also shows scarring and loss of vulvar architecture.

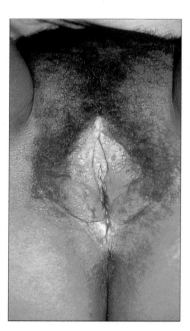

13.27 Lichen sclerosus. This patient complained of itching. Lichen simplex chronicus is superimposed on LS; biopsies confirmed LS and hyperkeratosis. There was no evidence of malignancy.

PAGET'S DISEASE

A biopsy should be taken of any solitary plaques (**13.28,13.29**) of oozy, crusted skin on the nipple or perianal area which grow slowly, do not itch, and do not resolve with topical steroids. While the diagnosis is usually suspected with a chronic unilateral nipple eczema, perineal lesions are often neglected for months or years. Several punch biopsies should be taken from representative areas, preferably the thickest part of a lesion rather than the base of an ulcer or erosion.

About 15% of patients have an associated carcinoma of an adjacent structure, such as the cervix, rectum, or urinary tract. The prognosis is worse in this group. In the remaining 85% of patients, tumor cells arise within the epidermis of the adjacent skin, probably from apocrine duct cells or pluripotential germinative cells.

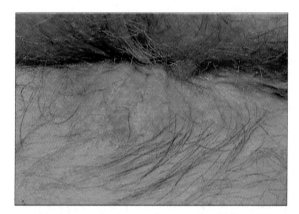

13.28 Extramammary Paget's disease. There is an asymmetric plaque of red, papillomatous skin with a white, oozy surface. There were no symptoms and the lesion did not respond to topical steroids.

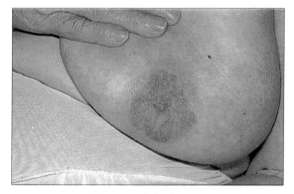

13.29 Paget's disease of the breast. An eczematous appearance is seen here, involving the entire areola and spreading onto the skin of the breast. This disorder should be suspected in any unilateral eruption affecting the areolar skin.

FURTHER READING

Gardner, S. S. and McKay, M. Seborrhea, psoriasis and the papulosquamous dermatoses. *Primary Care* 1989; **16**: 739–763.

McKay, M. Vulvodynia and pruritus vulvae. *Semin. Dermatol.* 1989; **8**: 40–47.

McKay, M. Vulvar dermatoses: common problems in dermatological and gynaecological practice. *Br. J. Clin. Prac.* 1990; **44**: 5–10.

McKay, M. Vulvar dermatoses. *Clin. Obstet. Gynecol.* 1991; **34**: 614–629.

McKay, M. Vulvitis and vulvovaginitis: cutaneous considerations. *Am. J. Obstet. Gynecol.* 1991; **165**: 1176–1182.

Pincus, S. H. Vulvar dermatoses and pruritus vulvae. *Dermatol. Clin.* 1992; **10**: 297–308.

Pincus, S. H. and McKay, M. Disorders of the female genitalia. In: *Dermatology in General Medicine.* 4th ed. Fitzpatrick, T. B., *et al.* (eds.): New York McGraw–Hill, 1993, pp.1463–1482.

Ridley, C. M. General dermatological conditions and dermatoses of the vulva. In: *The Vulva.* Ridley, C. M. (ed.) Edinburgh: Churchill Livingstone, 1988, pp.138–211.

Wilkinson, E., Ridley, C. M., McKay, M., *et al.* The ISSVD classification of vulvar nonneoplastic epithelial disorders and intraepithelial neoplasia. *Am. J. Dermatopathol.* 1991; **13**: 428–429.

ACKNOWLEDGEMENTS

Figure **13.1** is reproduced from G.M. Levene and S.K. Goolamali *Diagnostic Picture Tests in Dermatology* (Fig 127), Wolfe, London 1986. Figure **13.5** is reproduced from V.R. Tindall *Diagnostic Picture Tests in Dermatology* (Fig183), Wolfe, London 1987. Figures **13.6**, **13.26**, **13.28** and **13.29** are reproduced from C.M. Lawrence and N.H. Cox *Color Atlas and Text of Physical Signs in Dermatology* (Figs 8.11, 8.24, 8.16 and 8.15), Wolfe, London 1993.

14.
Vulvodynia and Pruritus Vulvae

Marilynne McKay

INTRODUCTION

Vulvodynia is the name given to chronic vulvar discomfort, especially if the patient complains of burning, stinging, irritation, or rawness[1]. Vulvodynia replaces the term 'burning vulva syndrome'. It is a different condition from pruritus vulvae – the latter means chronic itching, not burning (**14.1**) and the resultant scratching causes thickening of the skin. The patient with vulvar burning does not scratch, so there are rarely significant skin changes – erythema may be the only physical finding[2].

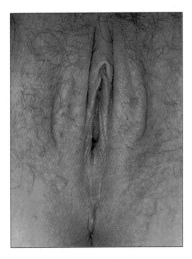

14.1 Patient with pruritus vulvae. Note the lichenification and excoriations caused by constant scratching of the skin. Patients with vulvar burning (vulvodynia) rarely have changes associated with scratching.

Vulvodynia can have many causes (**Table 14.1**), and a patient complaining of this symptom should be carefully evaluated[3,4]. The choice of therapy should depend on the patient's history and physical examination. No single treatment regimen is uniformly successful for all types of vulvodynia, and a careful history and physical examination are critical to selecting therapy. There is no 'overnight' or 'miracle' cure – even the correct medication may take weeks to improve the condition.

DIFFERENTIAL DIAGNOSIS

VULVAR DERMATOSES

These are cutaneous conditions likely to occur on the genitalia. They are now classified as 'non-neoplastic epithelial disorders' and the inaccurate term 'dystrophy' has been abolished[5] (*see Chapters 12 and 13*). Inflammation is present to some extent in all the dermatoses, and is thought to be important in maintaining the irritation of local nerve endings. The vulvar vestibule seems particularly susceptible, especially at the ostia of the vestibular glands, Bartholin's glands (at 5:00 and 7:00 in the posterior introitus), and Skene's periurethral glands. Pain and inflammation seem to be focused in these areas, and entry dyspareunia is persistent, even when there is minimal erythema on the rest of the vulva[6,7]. For this reason, trials of conservative therapy usually involve trying to decrease the inflammation for two to four months, in an attempt to see if the painful gland openings will recover spontaneously[8]. Fortunately, this is likely in at least 50% of cases, especially when the pain has been present for less than six months. Traumatic treatments (such as the carbon dioxide laser), which induce in-

| Vulvar dermatoses (non-neoplastic epithelial disorders) |
| Lichen sclerosus (LS) |
| Lichen simplex chronicus (LSC) |
| Steroid rebound dermatitis (SRD) |
| Psoriasis, seborrheic dermatitis |
| Erosive vulvitis, lichen planus (LP) |
| Irritant and allergic contact dermatitis |
| Atrophic vaginitis |
| Cyclic vulvovaginitis |
| Vulvar vestibulitis |
| Dyesthetic ('essential') vulvodynia |
| Pudendal neuralgia |

Table 14.1 Conditions Associated with Vulvodynia.

flammation, are now discouraged when the primary problem is one of vestibular pain[9,10].

'Subclinical' infection with human papillomavirus (HPV) was once thought to be a major factor in vulvar vestibulitis[11]. However, careful studies of vestibular tissue have not proven this to be the case[12,13].

Lichen Sclerosus

The whitened lesions of lichen sclerosus (LS, previously known as lichen sclerosus et atrophicus (LSA)) (**14.2**) may be asymptomatic, itch, or burn (*see Chapter 16*). Topical steroids have replaced testosterone and progesterone creams in the treatment of LS. (*See also Patient Information Sheets*, pp.182–183.)

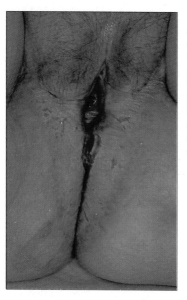

14.2. Lichen sclerosus. There is extensive involvement with peeling of the top layer of skin. Eroded areas may burn or sting when other areas of affected skin are not symptomatic.

Lichen Simplex Chronicus Secondary to Pruritus Vulvae

Lichen simplex chronicus (LSC) is the 'end-stage' cutaneous result of scratching (**14.3**). The patient may have started scratching because of itch due to recurrent *Candida* infections, tinea, or dermatitis. As a result, the patient's skin becomes thickened (lichenification). Some patients complain of burning or irritation only when they have excoriated and traumatized the top layer of the skin. Upon questioning, the skin is painful only when the patient has been scratching vigorously; otherwise, the primary symptom of LSC is itching[14,15]. (*See also Patient Information Sheet*, p. 184)

Management

When either LS or LSC have been confirmed by biopsy, the patient should be treated with the new superpotent Class 1 topical steroids (clobetasol propionate, halobetasol propionate, or betamethasone dipropionate in an optimized vehicle). Treatment should begin with a twice-daily application for one month, which is then tapered to daily for one month, and then to 'use only as needed'. Many patients obtain relief by applying treatment only once or twice weekly, or intermittently when symptoms occur. As there is a high risk of side-effects, Class 1 steroids should never be applied to vulvar skin without a confirmed diagnosis of LS or LSA.

Steroid Rebound Dermatitis

Steroid-rebound dermatitis (SRD) is iatrogenic and caused by the overuse of high-potency topical steroids on the skin of susceptible patients (**14.4**). It may be recognized as a fine-textured papular erythema with accentuated sebaceous glands. Patients often

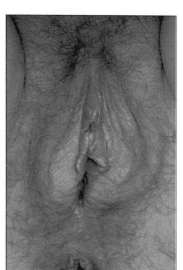

14.3 Lichen simplex chronicus (LSC). Leathery induration with accentuation of normal skin markings are the typical findings of LSC anywhere on the skin. The inner labia majora are often affected.

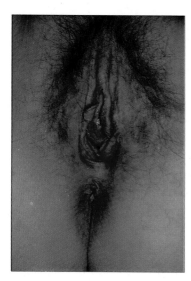

14.4 Steroid rebound dermatitis. Intense fine-textured papular erythema in the area where a Class 2 topical steroid (fluocinonide, 0.05% cream) had been applied for several months. The patient complained of burning, and was using the steroid cream to control the erythema.

complain of burning when the steroids are withdrawn, and the history usually confirms the diagnosis. Although high-potency Class 1 and 2 steroids are the usual offending agents, some patients may develop SRD with long-term use of relatively low-potency Class 4 medications.

Patients should be gradually weaned off the topical steroid by reducing the potency and frequency of use. *Candida* colonization is very common in these patients, and may account for flares of symptoms from time to time. As steroid is being used, there may be little vaginal discharge, but burning is intense and there may be significant swelling[3].

Psoriasis, Seborrheic Dermatitis

These conditions (**14.5**) may be recognized by typical lesions on the rest of the body (*see Chapter 13*). A vulvar biopsy can distinguish the dermatoses if differential diagnosis is a problem.

Erosive Vulvitis, Lichen Planus

This chronic problem (**14.6**) may be part of other dermatoses, such as the bullous diseases or lichen sclerosus. Lichen planus is often indicated by vaginal mucosal involvement, and lesions are therefore frequently found on the oral mucosa (*see Chapter 17*).

Irritant Dermatitis

If a patient complains of 'immediate stinging' when topical treatments are applied, this usually means that the normal barrier function of the skin has been compromised (**14.7**). Mucous membranes are very susceptible to drying, and vehicles containing astringents, alcohol, or propylene glycol will typically sting these areas. Local inflammation will also cause cutaneous sensitivity, no matter what the etiology (e.g. *Candida* infection, soaps, vigorous sexual intercourse). An irritant reaction does not mean that the patient is truly allergic to the substance, since the agent can often be applied to non-inflamed skin without problems.

The patient should be treated with mild topical steroids (hydrocortisone, 1%, preferably in an ointment base that contains few additives), or with easily obtainable bland emollients, such as milk compresses or vegetable shortening. Cool water or plastic ice-packs (wrapped in a rag) can help provide rapid relief of itching and swelling.

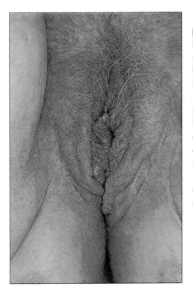

14.5 Extensive psoriasis of the labia majora with maceration and fissuring of the skin folds. The fissures (deep cracks) were painful and healed following treatment of the psoriasis with a mid-potency Class 4 topical steroid (triamcinolone acetonide, 0.1% ointment).

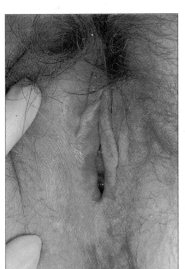

14.6 Lichen planus of the vulva with erosive vaginitis. The patient complained of burning and irritation with vaginal creams.

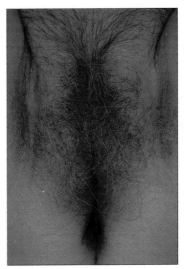

14.7 Irritant dermatitis to topical medication containing a relatively high concentration of propylene glycol, which was meant to be applied only once daily. The patient had been using it two or three times daily.

Allergic Contact Dermatitis

This is a cell-mediated allergic reaction on the patient's skin, which is produced at the point of contact with the allergen, every time that this contact occurs (**14.8, 14.9**). The rash does not begin immediately, but 24–48 hours after contact. The pattern of the rash provides a good clue to the diagnosis on exposed areas of the body, but in body folds, like the genitalia, the reaction may not be as obvious. Medications that cause allergic contact dermatitis in susceptible individuals include topicals containing the preservative ethylenediamine, the antibacterial neomycin, or the local anesthetic benzocaine. A suspected medication allergy can be tested using a 'use test'. This involves applying a possible allergen-containing medication to the forearm under an elastic bandage for 48 hours. Development of a rash may confirm the diagnosis. Caustic materials, such as powdered detergents, should not be tested in this way[15].

Atrophic Vaginitis

Uncomfortable dryness may be a problem for patients without adequate estrogenization of mucosal tissues, while the postmenopausal woman on estrogen replacement therapy may have an atypical presentation of *Candida* (**14.10**) with erythema and minimal discharge. Attempts to relieve the symptoms of irritation in either case may lead to 'overuse' problems with topical agents.

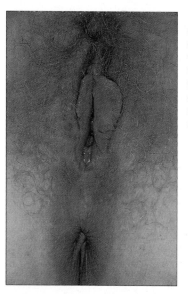

14.8 Allergic contact dermatitis of the vulva. The patient intermittently used a topical medication containing neomycin, to which she was allergic.

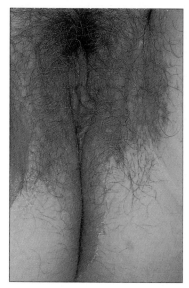

14.10 *Candida vulvovaginitis*, with typical erythema and peeling of the gluteal cleft and satellite pustules in the inguinal folds.

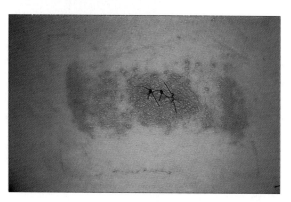

14.9 Allergic contact dermatitis. This was a reaction to an ointment containing neomycin, which had been applied under an adhesive plaster following excision of a nevus. The typical pattern where an allergen has touched the skin is a clue to diagnosis.

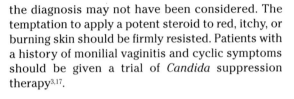

CYCLIC VULVOVAGINITIS

This is recurrent or recalcitrant vulvovaginitis, with or without typical, microscopically confirmed, monilial discharge (**14.11,14.12**). The patient usually confirms that she has occasional pain-free days, and/or that symptoms are worse at a particular time during the menstrual cycle. Dyspareunia is typically described as 'irritation afterwards'. Inflammatory symptoms suggest a local tissue hypersensitivity to *Candida*, with an exaggerated response to the presence of a very low concentration of the organism[16]. Although there is often swelling and itching, these patients rarely have a typical 'cottage-cheese' discharge and

the diagnosis may not have been considered. The temptation to apply a potent steroid to red, itchy, or burning skin should be firmly resisted. Patients with a history of monilial vaginitis and cyclic symptoms should be given a trial of *Candida* suppression therapy[3,17].

Treatment

The patient should be treated with low-dose, long-term anticandidals - either a vaginal cream or oral medication. A vaginal cream should be inserted every night for 10 days, followed by 1/2 applicator, Monday, Wednesday, and Friday, for two to four months. Maintenance therapy can be very helpful in some patients; vaginal cream should be used nightly for only the 3–5 days before menses each month.

Oral medications (e.g. ketoconazole or fluconazole) may be given daily for a short time (one to four weeks for ketoconazole) then tapered to an intermittent dosage (e.g. every other day) for two to four months. When using ketoconazole, liver function tests should be performed monthly. Fluconazole is metabolized by the kidneys, not the liver, and so is less toxic. Once- or twice-weekly dosages of fluconazole appear to be effective in suppressing *Candida* (*see also Chapter 15*).

VULVAR VESTIBULITIS

This is introital dyspareunia (pain upon entry of the vagina) with erythema and point tenderness to palpation at the openings of the minor vestibular glands, but without evidence of active infection (**14.13**). Intermittent symptoms are usually the result of local in-

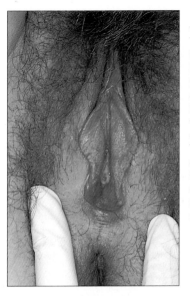

14.11 Cyclic vulvovaginitis. There is minimal involvement of the labia majora, but the minora are red and swollen. There is vaginal erythema, without a 'cottage cheese' discharge. The patient complained of burning and itching after coitus and monthly just before menses.

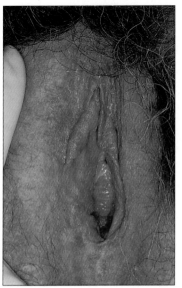

14.12 Cyclic vulvovaginitis. This postmenopausal patient was on estrogen replacement therapy. She complained of recurrent episodes of burning which were relieved by anticandidal vaginal creams. There is minimal vaginal discharge, but *Candida* was cultured from the erythematous area near the clitoris.

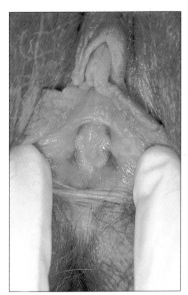

14.13 Vulvar vestibulitis. Erythema and point tenderness to cotton-tip palpation of the orifices of Bartholin's glands. Some tenderness is normal, and vulvar vestibulitis should be defined by dyspareunia that always occurs on entry.

flammation or *Candida*. Patients who can sometimes have coitus without pain have a much better prognosis than those who have had pain consistently for six months to a year. The patient with true vulvar vestibulitis has pain every time she attempts intercourse. In some patients, the pain may be severe enough to prevent coitus entirely.

Conservative Therapy

This consists in eliminating irritants and allergens and applying topical anti-inflammatory agents. If *Candida* has been documented, a *Candida* suppression regimen should be maintained for at least two months (*see above*). If the patient complains of irritation with topical agents, then systemic antifungals are indicated. A mid-strength topical steroid should be applied to the vulvar vestibule twice daily for one month, and then once daily. If the patient improves sufficiently to have coitus without pain even a few times, then conservative therapy should be continued, as gradual improvement is likely.

Vaginismus

Vaginismus may develop as a secondary problem to vestibulitis. Sometimes, treatment for vaginismus alone gives satisfactory results, probably because the vestibulitis has resolved spontaneously while the vaginismus has persisted. Treatment of vaginismus

is recommended before surgery. It will sometimes be effective and prevent the need for perineoplasty (*see below*). Even in cases where surgery is necessary, the patient will regain normal function more quickly afterwards if she has learned perineal relaxation techniques.

Other Therapy

Local injections of interferon have relieved pain in some cases, but usually the treatment has to be repeated. For patients with unremitting vestibular pain with coitus, surgery may be the best option. Removal of the painful crescent of skin at the posterior vestibule is successful in about 80% of cases. The technique is a modified perineoplasty, with an incision that includes the posterior hymenal ring and the vestibular tissue out to the perineal skin; posterior vaginal mucosa is advanced to cover the defect and the incision is closed (**14.14**). This procedure is considered by some to be the definitive therapy for vestibulitis[10]. The outcome is variable, however, and occasionally scar formation may prevent an entirely satisfactory result.

Another surgical treatment – with the carbon dioxide laser – has not been satisfactory for treating vestibulitis, possibly because of the prolonged healing time. In fact, the use of carbon dioxide laser

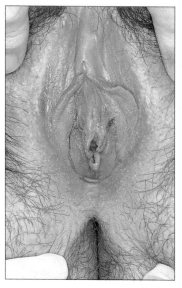

14.14 Surgical margins for posterior vestibulectomy. This operation is performed in cases of vulvar vestibulitis which do not respond to conservative therapy. The incision extends proximal to the posterior hymenal ring. The vaginal mucosa is mobilized and attached to the perineal skin, at the distal edge of the vestibular mucosal crescent, which is removed.

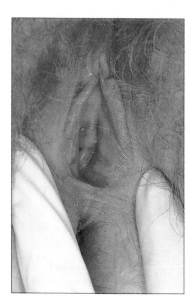

14.15 Vulvar vestibulitis. Extensive erythema and tenderness of posterior vestibular glands. This condition developed after treatment with a carbon dioxide laser.

for vulvar intraepithelial neoplasia has at times resulted in vulvar vestibulitis (**14.15**).

DYSESTHETIC ('ESSENTIAL') VULVODYNIA

Dysesthetic vulvodynia is chronic and continuous vulvar or vulvovaginal burning discomfort (**14.16**). It is often related to urethral syndrome or pudendal neuralgia. Older patients may have 'pelvic floor syndrome' due to the relaxation of the pelvic floor muscles with age. Some patients also complain of rectal discomfort or chronic low back pain. Younger patients with fibromyalgia, a poorly understood symptom complex characterized by musculoskeletal tenderness at various pressure points, may also have vulvar burning.

The condition responds to very low doses of systemic antidepressant therapy, such as amitriptyline, nortriptyline, or trazodone, though fluoxetine has not been as effective[18]. These medications have been helpful in other types of dysesthesias (e.g. postzoster neuralgia), but should be instituted with caution. In the elderly patient, treatment should begin slowly at a low dose. For example, amitriptyline should be started at 10–20mg at bedtime, and increased by 10mg weekly to a maximum dosage of 50–75mg at bedtime.

REFERENCES

1 Burning vulva syndrome: report of the ISSVD task force. *J. Reprod. Med.* 1984; **29**: 457.
2 McKay, M. Vulvodynia versus pruritus vulvae. *Clin. Obstet. Gynecol.* 1985; **28**: 123–133.
3 McKay, M. Vulvodynia: diagnostic patterns. *Dermatol. Clin.* 1992; 10: 423–433.
4 McKay, M. Vulvodynia: a multifactorial problem. *Arch. Dermatol.* 1989; **125**: 256–262.
5 Wilkinson, E., Ridley, C. M., McKay, M., *et al.* The ISSVD classification of vulvar nonneoplastic epithelial disorders and intraepithelial neoplasia. *Am. J. Dermatopathol.* 1991; **13**: 428–429.
6 Friedrich, E. G. Jr. Vulvar vestibulitis syndrome. *J. Reprod. Med.* 1987; **32**: 110–114.
7 McKay, M., Frankman, O., Horowitz, B. J., *et al.* Vulvar vestibulitis and vestibular papillomatosis: report of the ISSVD committee on vulvodynia. *J. Reprod. Med.* 1991; **36**: 413–415.
8 Pyka, R. E., Wilkinson, E. J., Friedrich, E. G. Jr., *et al.* The histopathology of vulvar vestibulitis syndrome. *Internat. J. Gynecol. Pathol.* 1988; **7**: 249–257.
9 Friedrich, E. G. Jr. Therapeutic studies on vulvar vestibulitis. *J. Reprod. Med.* 1988; **33**: 514–518.
10 Marinoff, S. C. and Turner, M. L. C. Vulvar vestibulitis syndrome. *Dermatol. Clin.* 1992; **10**: 435–444.
11 Growdon, W. A., Fu, Y. S., Lebherz, T. B., *et al.* Pruritic vulvar squamous papillomatosis: evidence for human papillomavirus etiology. *Obstet. Gynecol.* 1985; **66**: 564–568.
12 Moyal-Barracco, M., Leibowitch, M., and Orth, G. Vestibular papillae of the vulva. Lack of evidence for human papillomavirus etiology. *Arch. Dermatol.* 1990; **126**: 1594–1598.
13 Bergeron, C., Ferenczy, A., Richart, R. M., *et al.* Micropapillomatosis labialis appears unrelated to human papillomavirus. *Obstet. Gynecol.* 1990; **76**: 281–286.
14 Pincus, S. H. Vulvar dermatoses and pruritus vulvae. *Dermatol. Clin.* 1992; **10**: 297–308.
15 McKay, M. Vulvitis and vulvovaginitis: cutaneous considerations. *Am. J. Obstet. Gynecol.* 1991; **165**: 1176–1182.
16 Witkin, S. S., Jeremias, J., and Ledger, W. J. A localized vaginal allergic response in women with recurrent vaginitis. *J. Allergy Clin. Immunol.* 1988; **81**: 412–416.
17 Sobel, J. Recurrent vulvovaginal candidiasis: a prospective study of the efficacy of maintenance ketoconazole therapy. *N. Engl. J. Med.* 1986; **315**: 1455–1458.
18 McKay, M. Dysesthetic ('essential') vulvodynia: treatment with amitriptyline. *J. Reprod. Med.* 1993; **38**: 9–13.

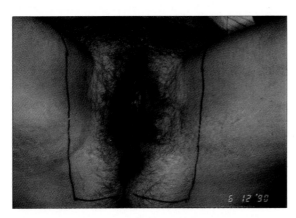

14.16 Dysesthetic vulvodynia. The patient complained of unremitting burning in the area supplied by the pudendal nerve (outlined by marking pen). This area was hypersensitive to light touch when compared to the rest of the skin.

ACKNOWLEDGMENT

Figure **14.16** has been reproduced by kind permission of Maria L. Chanco Turner.

15.
Infectious Vaginitis

M. John Hare

INTRODUCTION

Symptoms suggestive of vaginal infection are one of the most common reasons for a woman to consult her doctor. Most cases are simple and uncomplicated and respond well to a single course of appropriate treatment. However, a few cases develop into chronic problems, with difficulty in diagnosis, multiple treatments, complete disruption of the normal physiologic and microbiologic vaginal environment, and often chronic psychologic and psychosexual disorders (*see Chapter 14*). These cases are difficult to control and may require a multidisciplinary input, including from family physicians, gynecologists, genitourinary physicians, microbiologists, dermatologists, psychologists, and psychosexual counsellors. The best strategy for avoiding such chronic problems is to diagnose and treat accurately the initial presenting complaint.

PHYSIOLOGY OF THE LOWER GENITAL TRACT

The physiologic function of the vagina is to act as a channel between the uterine cervix and the vulva for the purposes of reproduction. Fertilization is achieved by penovaginal coitus, with deposition of spermatozoa close to the cervix. Adequate lubrication is essential and is achieved by:

- A transudate of serous fluid through the vaginal wall. During sexual excitement, the blood vessels surrounding the vagina become engorged, and the rate of production of fluid is increased.
- Discharge produced by the uterus and uterine cervix. Although vaginal discharge is normally insignificant in quantity, it may increase to a noticeable level if the cervix is infected or covered in columnar cell ectopy.
- Secretion from Bartholin's glands. In animals, these glands produce pheromones for sexual attraction and during sexual excitement, but they have a much reduced function in the human.

NORMAL VAGINAL DISCHARGE

The quantity of discharge accepted as normal will vary from woman to woman. Complaints will tend to be about an increase in the volume of discharge and/ or a change in its characteristics.

During the reproductive years, vaginal discharge is white and fairly thick, though it thins out during sexual excitement. Under the microscope, it is seen to contain a large proportion of superficial squamous cells with small pyknotic nuclei. These stain pink with Papanicolaou reagents. Döderlein's bacilli (lactobacilli) are common, and there may be a variety of other bacteria. In mid-cycle, leukocytes are rare, but become more common immediately before the start of or after the end of the menstrual cycle.

Immediately after birth and for the following few months, the condition of the vagina is similar to that during the reproductive years. This is in response to high maternal estrogen levels at birth. During this time, heavy vaginal discharge may be noted. In the prepubertal and postmenopausal years, the volume of discharge tends to be less, and postmenopausal dryness is often a complaint. The predominant cells seen under the microscope are parabasal and intermediate in type. They have proportionately larger nuclei than seen in superficial cells, and the nuclei stain blue with Papanicolaou reagents. Leukocytes may be common, and a variety of microorganisms are seen on staining.

In pregnancy, navicular cells predominate – they are a type of intermediate cell. Exogenous hormones will tend to modify the cellular pattern. For example, unopposed estrogen given after hysterectomy will tend to result in mature cells, while progesterone-dominated oral contraceptives will tend to produce a pattern of intermediate-type cells.

Vaginal acidity (pH) varies with age and hormonal changes. During the reproductive years, the vagina is acid (pH 4.5 or less) due to the metabolism of glycogen in the cells of the vaginal walls. Before puberty, and after the menopause, the pH level is close to neutral.

MICROBIOLOGY

The vagina contains a high density of a large variety of microorganisms. For more than a century, it was thought that the vagina contained a simple and stable flora dominated by Döderlein's bacilli. This theory is no longer tenable, and the vaginal flora is probably both varied and mobile. As well as lactobacilli and bifidobacteria, commonly isolated organisms include those listed in **Table 15.1**.

With very few exceptions, such as *Treponema pallidum, Neisseria gonorrhoeae, Chlamydia trachomatis*, and possibly *Trichomonas vaginalis*, almost any microorganism may be found in the healthy vagina. It is diagnostically important not to attempt to define normal vaginal flora without taking into account the age and sexual experience of the woman concerned.

Anaerobes Bacteroides Peptostreptococci Gardnerella Mobiluncus Clostridia Actinomyces Aerobes Streptococci Staphylococci Micrococci Enterobacteriaceae Pseudomonadaceae Mycoplasma Ureaplasma Yeasts	**Table 15.1** **Normal Vaginal** **Microflora –** **Common** **Microbial** **Isolates.**

CLINICAL EXAMINATION OF THE VAGINA

Vaginal infection cannot be diagnosed properly without a thorough clinical examination. For this, the physician needs an examination room with a suitable couch, a good light, and privacy. A female chaperone is essential for a male physician performing a vaginal examination.

Although the idealist might wish to approach every case in the same way (and there is academic merit in such an argument), epidemiologic, social and, not least, economic factors will dictate that patients are managed differently, according to the way in which they present.

The teenage prostitute presenting in the genitourinary medicine clinic and the middle-aged housewife and mother presenting to her family physician may both have sexually transmitted infections. However, the former will always be screened for these, while the latter will usually not be. To screen for all possible infections in every case would consume vast amounts of resources for very little gain;

not to do so will allow a small number of significant infections to go unreported.

The decision as to how far to go with laboratory tests in individual cases must be based on sensitive but thorough history taking, epidemiologic knowledge, and common sense. Although not essential, a colposcope does make vaginal examination easier, as there are some situations in which a magnified view of the vagina is helpful.

EXAMINATION TECHNIQUE

The vulva and vestibule are first inspected for signs of infection and other disease, and the inguinal areas are palpated for clinically apparent lymph nodes. An unlubricated (or water-lubricated) bivalve vaginal speculum (Cusco pattern) (**15.1**) is passed into the vagina and opened to expose the uterine cervix. If the patient's legs are supported in stirrups or foot rests, the speculum is best inserted handle downwards. However, if the patient is lying flat on a couch, the speculum is best inserted handle upwards.

The lateral vaginal walls are now exposed, together with the fornices. Vaginal discharge may have collected in the posterior blade of the speculum; **Table 15.2** lists the tests that should be performed on a sample of this discharge. The vagina is then cleared of discharge, and the cervix is wiped clean. If there is a significant risk of sexually transmitted infection, tests for pathogens (*N. gonorrhoeae, C. trachomatis*, and possibly herpesvirus) are performed on smears taken from the endocervix. A cervical smear is usually stained by the Papanicolaou method, to test both for the presence of premalignant change

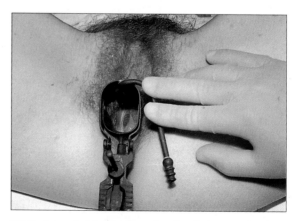

15.1 A vaginal speculum in place. This speculum has a smoke extractor incorporated into it to allow operation on the cervix with diathermy or laser.

pH (acidity)
Wet film preparation, emulsified in saline and in
    10% KCl
Gram stain
Amine ('sniff') test
Culture
    Candida and other yeasts
    Trachomatis vaginalis
    Mycoplasma and *Ureaplasma* (if required)
General bacterial culture

Table 15.2 Investigations Performed on Vaginal Discharge.

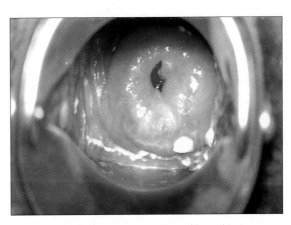

15.2 A normal cervix seen through a colposcope.

(cervical intraepithelial neoplasia, CIN) and for cellular marks of infection.

The visible portion of the vagina and the cervix are now carefully inspected, under magnification if a colposcope is available (**15.2**). A washout with normal saline may be necessary to obtain a proper view, and if premalignant change of the cervix or vagina is suspected, colposcopic examination should be repeated after application of 5% acetic acid.

The inspection is continued by gradual withdrawal and partial closure of the speculum, which will reveal the previously concealed parts of the anterior and posterior walls of the vagina. The overall picture of the vaginal wall is noted, together with specific features such as ulcers, warty lesions, or keratin plaques.

As the speculum is finally withdrawn, it will have 'milked' the urethra to reveal any discharge. This discharge may need to be tested for infection. Skene's and Bartholin's glands should be palpated and the entrances to their ducts inspected for discharge. Finally, a bimanual examination should be carried out, with full palpation of the upper pelvic organs.

SYMPTOMS OF VAGINAL INFECTION

The symptoms of vaginal infection are often associated and/or confused with symptoms related to associated areas. The commonest presenting symptoms are an increase in vaginal discharge, vaginal soreness, and vaginal odor, with or without discharge.

Vaginal Discharge

This is likely to be due to a vaginal condition, bloodstained fluid is more likely to be related to the cervix or uterus. The following characteristics should be noted:

- Color – clear, yellow, green, bloodstained, brown, or black;
- Amount – assessed by the need to use sanitary pads or other protection;
- Smell – offensive or non-offensive;
- Irritancy – presence or non-presence.

Vaginal Soreness

This may be a symptom by itself, or may be related to tampon use or sexual intercourse. Soreness on intercourse (dyspareunia) may be superficial (at the start of penetration) or deep (related to deep penetration only). Deep dyspareunia tends to be related to pelvic conditions other than vaginitis. Dysuria may also be a presenting symptom.

Vaginal Odor, with or without Discharge

This may be worse during particular times, such as menstruation, and may be further worsened by sexual intercourse.

SPECIFIC CONDITIONS

VAGINAL THRUSH (CANDIDOSIS, MONILIASIS, VAGINAL CANDIDIASIS)

This condition commonly presents as vulvar and vaginal itching, with or without discharge. If a discharge is present, it is typically yellow-white and has a thick and cheesy consistency. The condition develops most commonly in the week preceding menstruation, and symptoms are worse when the genital area is both warm and confined, for example, in bed at night or when wearing tights or clothes made of synthetic materials. An offensive odor is unusual, but dyspareunia and dysuria are common.

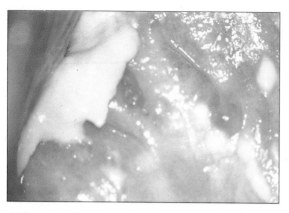

15.3 Vaginal candidiasis. Thick plaques of curdy discharge typical of vaginal thrush.

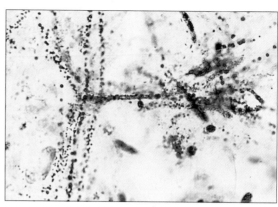

15.4 Vaginal candidiasis. Gram-stained film of vaginal discharge showing spores and hyphae of *Candida albicans*.

On clinical examination, the vulva and vestibule are seen to be obviously inflamed, often with fissuring and erosion due to scratching. On passage of a speculum, thick plaques of curdy discharge are seen on the vaginal walls and the cervix (**15.3**). The vaginal pH is less than 4.5. On examination of a wet preparation or a Gram-stained film, budding yeast cells and hyphal forms may be seen (**15.4**). Culture can be carried out using selective media, and a specific latex agglutinate test is available for the identification of *Candida albicans*.

Causative Organisms

Most cases (85%) of clinical vaginal thrush are caused by *C. albicans*, but symptomatic disease has also been attributed to *C. tropicalis* and *C. paropsilosis*. *Candida glabrata*, previously known as *Torulopsis glabrata*, is said to account for 5% of vaginal fungal infections, but these are at the milder end of the clinical scale and rarely give rise to florid symptoms and signs.

Pathogenesis

Candida albicans is found in the mouth and the intestinal tract of a substantial proportion of the normal population. It should probably also be regarded as a normal inhabitant of the female genital tract, occurring in the vagina in up to 10% of non-pregnant women and up to 40% of pregnant women. Thus, it may be argued that the development of the disease process represents a failure of the host's defense mechanisms, though allergy is thought to be an important factor in some cases, and some strains are more virulent than others.

Predisposing Factors

Although many factors are claimed to be precipitating factors for vaginal thrush, definitive evidence is hard to find. Certainly, broad-spectrum antibiotic treatment and coexisting diabetes mellitus appear to be definite associations. Probably in response to the changed immune status, vaginal thrush does appear to be more common in pregnancy, with an incidence of up to 30% being reported. The relationship with oral contraceptive use is controversial, with some authors claiming an increased risk of development of thrush, especially when high-estrogen combined pills are used. This could be related to the immunocompromised state caused by oral contraception. Women with any immunodepressed state are prone to develop this infection.

Treatment

Two groups of drugs, the polyene antifungals and the imidazoles, are the first-line options for treatment. Pessaries are the commonest formulation used, but vaginal cream and impregnated tampons are also used. In severe pruritus, a mixture of an antifungal agent and weak hydrocortisone cream is soothing when applied to the vulva. Nystatin is the usually available polyene antifungal, normally given as vaginal tablets (pessaries). However, patient compliance is often poor, as nystatin has the disadvantage that it must be used for 14 consecutive nights. It also stains underclothes.

Local imidazole derivatives used are clotrimazole, miconazole, econazole, and isoconazole, which are all available as single-application treatments. The first three may also be used for longer courses. Oral medication (ketoconazole, itraconazole, and fluconazole) is best regarded as second-line treatment for vaginal thrush. Ketoconazole may be hepatotoxic, and *C. tropicalis* is resistant to fluconazole.

Recurrent Thrush

Due to the ubiquitous presence of *Candida* and its complex relationship with its host, recurrent thrush is common and may be difficult to eradicate. In such cases, it is vital to confirm the diagnosis by microbiologic culture and to exclude other causes of the symptoms and signs. Precipitating and predisposing causes must be sought and eliminated wherever possible, and the patient encouraged to wear cotton rather than synthetic clothing and to practise good hygiene.

The role of sexual transmission in vaginal thrush is debatable. While most authorities would not consider investigating and treating a sexual partner at a first attack, this should be done if the condition is recurrent. The patient's own bowel has also been considered as a source of reinfection, though there is no clinical evidence that attempting to clear the bowel of *Candida* improves the outcome. Evidence for an underlying immune deficiency should also be sought.

For those for whom no cause of recurrence can be found, relief may be provided by intermittent prophylactic treatment. Single treatments are given once per month, at either the start or finish of menstruation. Such treatments have been beneficial using either vaginal imidazole or oral preparations. *(See also cyclic vulvovaginitis, Chapter 14).*

TRICHOMONIASIS

This condition classically presents as an acute vaginitis, with a profuse malodorous discharge and associated soreness, dysuria, and dyspareunia. On examination, the vaginal walls are seen to have a typical punctate appearance, the so-called 'strawberry' vagina (**15.5**). However, this description was coined before the recognition of bacterial vaginosis as a clinical entity, and a similar appearance also occurs with this condition. Trichomonal vaginosis and bacterial vaginosis commonly coexist in the florid clinical situations described above. 'Pure' trichomonal vaginitis is often a much milder condition. The vaginal pH is greater than 4.5, usually 5.5–6.0. The diagnosis can almost always be made in the clinic upon examination of a film of discharge emulsified in normal saline – typical motile organisms of *T. vaginalis* are seen (**15.6**). The organism's

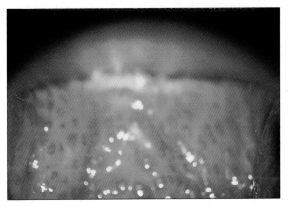

15.5 Trichomoniasis. Strawberry vaginitis, typical of trichomonal infection is shown, although a bacterial vaginosis may result in a similar appearance.

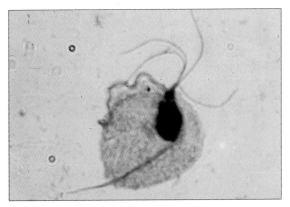

15.6 *Trichomonas vaginalis* in a fresh wet preparation. This organism will be vigorously motile.

presence can be confirmed by culture in selective media.

Causative Organism

The causative organism is *T. vaginalis*, a large single-celled flagellate. It has a very distinctive appearance, especially when it is moving. It should be remembered that routine cytology staining by the Papanicolaou method may be unreliable, with false positive rates of up to 48%. If symptoms and signs are not present, and the diagnosis has not been confirmed by another method, cytologic diagnoses should be regarded as unproven.

Treatment

Metronidazole remains the almost invariable treatment for this condition. The success rates of 98% obtained by Keighley in her early work in a women's prison are still usual. Treatments can be tailored to the patient's need, lasting between one and seven days. Relative resistance to metronidazole has been reported in a small number of cases, but treatment failure is more likely to be due to poor compliance, malabsorption, or reinfection. In most such cases, re-treatment with a seven-day course at double dosage, or the use of rectal or parenteral preparations of the same drug, should suffice. Povidone–iodine may be used as a support measure for treatment with metronidazole, and is available as vaginal pessaries, vaginal gel, or vaginal douche.

Recurrent Trichomoniasis

In cases of persistent failure of treatment or recurrence, the male partner(s) should be investigated. Evidence suggests that in most cases, *T. vaginalis* is not permanently harbored by the male sexual partners of women with trichomoniasis, but colonizes the male genitalia for only a week or so after intercourse with an infected female. In most cases, a course of metronidazole for the female partner followed by abstinence, while awaiting a test of cure, will be effective against reinfection. However, in a few cases, the male is a long-term reservoir of infection – which sometimes causes urethritis. Thus, if the woman fails to respond to standard treatment, her partner(s) should be examined and treated.

BACTERIAL VAGINOSIS

This term is used to describe a syndrome characterized by a malodorous vaginal discharge and raised vaginal pH. A typical symptom is a vaginal discharge that is excessive, stains clothes green or yellow, and has an offensive odor, often likened to the smell of fish. The odor is particularly noticeable after sexual intercourse, when alkaline semen has been deposited in the vagina. It is often a chronic condition. Irritation, dyspareunia and dysuria are uncommon symptoms. The clinical appearance of the discharge is variable; clinical inflammation of the vagina and surrounding areas is unusual.

Causative Organisms

Gardnerella vaginalis was once thought to be the sole causative agent, but it is now known that *Mobiluncus* and *Bacteroides* species play a more important role. Bacterial vaginosis must be considered a disorder of the normal microbiologic flora of the vagina. A dramatic decline in the number of Döderlein's bacilli (lactobacilli) allows other organisms to multiply,

especially anaerobes. In the past, the disease has been referred to as non-specific vaginitis, *Haemophilus vaginalis* vaginitis, *Corynebacterium vaginitis*, *Gardnerella* vaginitis, and anaerobic vaginosis. All these terms have been discarded in favor of bacterial vaginosis: 'bacterial' because both aerobes and anaerobes may be involved; and 'vaginosis' rather than vaginitis, because there is no great release of white blood cells. Purists may argue with some justification that the correct nomenclature should be vaginal bacteriosis – and this change may yet come. However, the diagnosis of this condition is reached by assessment of the clinical picture, not by the culture of a particular organism.

Diagnosis

The diagnosis of bacterial vaginosis rests on four factors:
- A vaginal pH greater than 4.5.
- A homogenic, thin, vaginal discharge.
- A positive amine ('sniff') test. A small amount of discharge is placed on a microscope slide and a drop of 10% potassium chloride is added to it. A fish-like amine odor is noticed immediately, similar to that produced by the action of the relatively alkaline seminal fluid on the vaginal contents.
- The presence of 'clue cells' in wet or Gram-stained vaginal preparations. Clue cells are epithelial cells covered in bacteria, usually curved rods. The appearance is very striking, sometimes giving a 'scratched edge' appearance to the cells (**15.7**).

As well as these features, a large number of micro-organisms are often seen in the background in wet or Gram-stained smears of vaginal secretion. These are usually curved, motile rods of the *Mobiluncus* species. Simplified diagnostic techniques are described by Sonnex (1995)[1]. Bacterial culture does not play a part

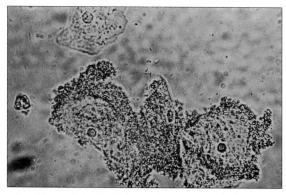

15.7 Bacterial vaginosis. 'Clue cells' typical of bacterial vaginosis seen in a wet preparation.

in the diagnosis of bacterial vaginosis, though it may be needed to exclude other pathogens. In particular, the isolation of *G. vaginalis* on bacterial culture is not diagnostic of bacterial vaginosis.

Treatment

As no specific microorganism is responsible for the clinical syndrome of bacterial vaginosis, it is not surprising that no treatment is 100% effective. Metronidazole is the most commonly prescribed antibiotic, with a success rate of over 90% for seven-day courses. If this fails, ampicillin (or amoxycillin) is the drug of second choice. Clindamycin is highly effective, and may be given as a vaginal cream. Other vaginal preparations, such as triple-sulpha and povidone–iodine, may also be used.

Recurrent Bacterial Vaginosis

As might be anticipated from the nature of the disease, recurrent attacks are common. Although sexual transmission of the relevant organism is possible, the treatment of male partners does not appear to be helpful. Separation of partners, by condom use or abstinence, may be worthwhile. Attention should be paid to hygiene, and possibly a change in contraceptive practice.

Vaginal acidification or attempts to colonize the vagina with lactobacilli (in yogurt) are not effective. Recently, the presence of bacterial vaginosis organisms in pregnancy has been associated with late miscarriage and premature labor. Trials are underway to assess whether or not antibiotic treatment of the organisms will reduce the risk of these events.

VAGINAL WARTS 'CONDYLOMATOUS VAGINITIS'

Genital warts may affect the uterine cervix (**15.8**, **15.9**), vagina, vulva, and perineal area. The vagina is less commonly involved, with 15% of typical genital warts found at this site, usually with vulvar or cervical lesions as well. Vaginal intraepithelial neoplasia is usually associated with the development of multisite lower genital intraepithelial neoplasia, or it may be a residual lesion left behind after hysterectomy for cervical intraepithelial neoplasia. Isolated vaginal warts do not require biopsy unless the appearance is atypical. They can be treated by cytotoxic therapy (podophyllin), chemical destruction (trichloroacetic acid), or physical destruction (loop diathermy, laser cryotherapy) or excision.

Microscopic wart virus infection of the whole vagina has been described, and named 'condylomatous vaginitis'. To the naked eye, the vagina simply ap-

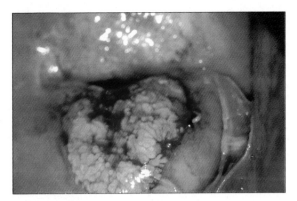

15.8 Papilliferous wart on the uterine cervix.

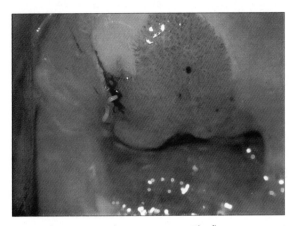

15.9 Flat wart on the uterine cervix. The flat wart is more common than the papilliferous wart.

pears roughened, but under colposcopic examination 'microwarts' are seen with their typical papillary loop appearance. Patients with this condition sometimes complain of therapy-resistant vaginal soreness, dryness, and frequent dyspareunia. If symptoms suggest that treatment is needed, the patient should be asked if particularly troublesome areas can be identified which can be subjected to local destructive therapy[2]. Failing this, symptomatic remedies are all that can be offered.

PREPUBERTAL AND POSTMENOPAUSAL VAGINITIS

From a few months after birth until puberty and after the menopause, estrogen stimulation of the vagina is low. The walls are thin and the cells lining the vagina are immature and contain little glycogen. Lactobacilli are absent, and the vagina is colonized by a mixed bacterial flora. The pH is about the neutral level.

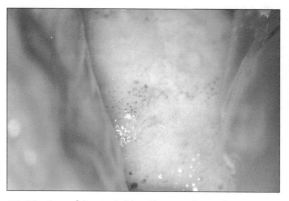

15.10 Atrophic vaginitis. Changes of atrophic vaginitis seen in a postmenopausal woman. A degree of vaginal wall prolapse is present.

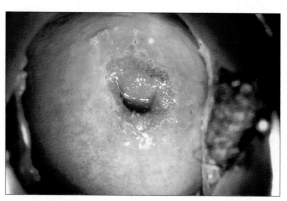

15.11 Columnar cell ectopy. A small area of columnar cell ectopy surrounds the cervical os on a normal cervix.

Prepubertal Girls

In the prepubertal girl, vaginal infection is usually caused by irritation from a foreign body, and a careful search must be made for one. Sexual assault must be considered as a possible vehicle for infection and, if appropriate, tests should be taken for *C. trachomatis*, *N. gonorrhoeae* and *T. vaginalis*. Gastrointestinal infections can infect the genital tract, including the roundworm, *Enterobius vermicularis*. The traditional method of detecting this parasite is by placing sticky tape across the perineum.

Postmenopausal Women

Vaginitis in the postmenopausal woman is usually due to estrogen depletion. At the menopause, the whole of the vagina loses its overall appearance of rugae, and becomes less elastic (**15.10**). Gross thinning of the epithelial layers results in a vaginal epithelium that is prone to infection and tears easily. The symptoms of atrophic postmenopausal vaginitis include discharge (which may be bloodstained), soreness, and dyspareunia. This condition may be the sole reason for postmenopausal bleeding, though other causes must be sought for this presentation, especially malignant change. If atrophic vaginitis is the definitive diagnosis, treatment is by local or systemic estrogen administration. In severe cases, bacterial culture and appropriate antibiotic therapy may also be needed.

CERVICAL AND OTHER VAGINAL LESIONS CAUSING VAGINAL DISCHARGE

Lesions or changes on the uterine cervix may cause vaginal discharge. As the squamocolumnar junction may be on the vagina rather than the vaginal portion of the cervix, the vagina may be included in these changes. Before reaching any conclusion about the cause and nature of vaginal disease, the uterine cervix must be seen clearly in a good light. The result of a current or recent cervical smear must be available at the time of treatment or soon after. Any suspicious appearance of the cervix should be investigated by colposcopy and biopsy, as cytology alone may not detect cervical carcinoma. Blood and necrotic debris may obscure the diagnostic features of malignant change in such slides.

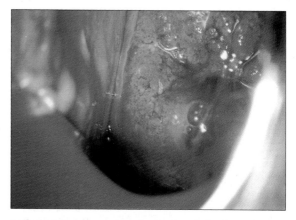

15.12 Columnar cell ectopy. The whole of the uterine cervix is covered in columnar cell ectopy. This will result in excessive but physiological vaginal discharge.

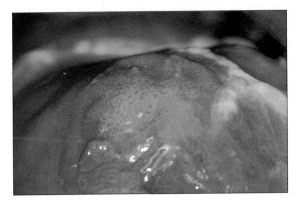

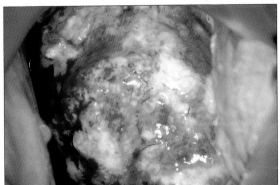

15.13 Vaginal adenosis. Columnar cell ectopy on the anterior lip of the uterine cervix and extending onto the vagina. This condition is known as vaginal adenosis.

15.14 Invasive cervical carcinoma.

COLUMNAR CELL ECTOPY

Columnar cell ectopy, sometimes misnamed as a 'cervical erosion', is the presence of visible columnar epithelium on the vaginal portion of the uterine cervix (**15.11**). In its exaggerated form (**15.12**), it extends out onto the upper portion of the vagina, and is then referred to as vaginal adenosis (**15.13**). The use of the bivalve speculum increases the impression of cervical ectopy by forcing open the canal of the parous cervix; if the blades are allowed to close slightly after opening fully, the area of change will decrease to its proper size.

Columnar cell ectopy is a normal feature on the uterine cervix. It is prominent at birth, and increases again at the menarche when hormones cause the lips of the cervix to evert. Columnar epithelium subjected to the vaginal environment (especially low acidity) undergoes the process of squamous metaplasia, in which it is replaced by metaplastic squamous epithelium. Such change may be delayed by hormones (especially oral contraception) and by pregnancy.

Columnar epithelium is prone to non-specific infection, which may cause excessive discharge. Rarely, if this cannot be controlled by local or systemic treatment, the area of ectopy should be destroyed using cryotherapy or diathermy. Healing usually results in the development of squamous epithelium at the site, especially if an acid environment is maintained during healing.

CERVICAL INFECTIONS

Cervical infections may be due to vaginal organisms (ectocervix), while infections of the endocervical canal are more likely to be sexually transmitted. If endocervicitis is suspected, tests must be taken for *N. gonorrhoeae* and *C. trachomatis*. Cervicitis due to herpesvirus hominis may also be present; it usually occurs, but not always, in association with vulvar herpetic lesions.

CERVICAL CARCINOMA

Cervical carcinoma may also cause vaginal discharge (**15.14**). As stated above, the use of cytology alone to investigate a suspicious cervical appearance may result in a cervical carcinoma being overlooked. The diagnostic features of malignant change may be obscured by blood and debris in cytology and therefore missed.

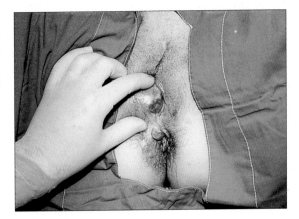

15.15 Swollen Bartholin's gland, seen before surgical drainage.

INFECTIONS OF BARTHOLIN'S GLAND

Bartholin's gland may be infected by various organisms, and once infection has occurred, it may follow a classical path of development. In the young and nulliparous woman, sexually transmitted agents play a major part in the genesis of infection – either *C. trachomatis* or *N. gonorrhoeae* may be implicated. Swelling of the gland (**15.15**) and consequent blockage of the duct may lead to secondary infection, first by aerobic organisms and then by anaerobic species. At this stage, an abscess may form within the gland and duct. If the gland does not burst or drain, the infection may resolve spontaneously, leaving a sterile fluid filled swelling - a Bartholin's cyst.

In the older woman, with a perineum distorted by childbirth and with a greater risk of bacterial vaginosis, a primary infection of Bartholin's gland may occur with resident aerobic or anaerobic organisms. Gland infections may lead to abscess formation. Duct infections without gland involvement will lead to cyst formation with clear fluid collecting in the gland.

Management
The management of a swelling or inflammation of Bartholin's gland will depend on the clinical assessment of the stage of the disease.

- A swollen, tender, and non-fluctuant Bartholin's gland suggests infection without abscess formation. Genital cultures should be taken, including any secretion draining from Bartholin's ducts, and appropriate broad-spectrum antibiotic treatment should be given.
- An acutely tender fluctuant gland suggests that abscess formation has occurred; in this case drainage is required.
- A non-tender, but swollen and fluctuant gland suggests cyst formation without the presence of active infection. The treatment for such lesions is marsupialization, in which a new aperture of about 1cm length for the gland is created, just outside the hymenal ring, and the skin edges are sutured to the cyst edges to maintain drainage *(see Chapter 20)*.

Recurrent cysts or abscess of Bartholin's gland are best treated by excision.

INFECTION OF SKENE'S GLAND

This gland is usually involved in cases of gonococcal or chlamydial urethritis, and in such cases will respond to the appropriate antibiotic therapy (**15.16**). In the older woman, chronic infection with non-sexually transmitted organisms can occur, often with blockage of the gland. As well as antibiotic therapy, probing of the gland may be necessary to achieve drainage. In extreme cases, the gland may need to be destroyed by diathermy.

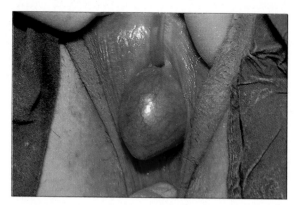

15.16 Grossly swollen cyst of Skene's gland.

REFERENCES
1. Sonnex, C. The amine test: a simple rapid inexpensive method for diagnosing bacterial vaginosis. *Br. J. Obst. Gynecol.* 1995; **102**: 160–161.
2. Rulander, E., Eriksson, A. and von Schoultz, B. Wart virus infection of cervix uteri and vagina with atypical cervical cytology. In: Mårdh, P.A. and Taylor-Robinson, D. *Bacterial Vaginosus.* Stockholm: Almqvist and Wiksell International, 1984, pp223–226.

FURTHER READING
Berger, G. S. and Weström, J. V. (eds.) *Pelvic Inflammatory Disease.* New York: Raven Press, 1992.
Eschenbach, D. A., *et al.* Diagnosis and clinical manifestations of bacterial vaginosis. *Am. J. Obstet. Gynecol.* 1988; **158**: 819–828.
Hare, M. J. (ed.) *Genital Tract Infection in Women.* Edinburgh: Churchill Livingstone, 1988, pp.199–215.
McGregor, J. A. and Hammill, H. A. Contraception and sexually transmitted diseases: interactions and opportunities. *Am. J. Obstet. Gynecol.* 1993; **168**: 2033–2041.
Pastorek, J. G. (ed.) *Obstetric and Gynecologic Infectious Disease.* New York: Raven Press, 1993.
Washington, A. E., *et al.* Preventing pelvic inflammatory disease. *J.A.M.A.* 1991; **266**: 2574–2580.

16.
Vulvar Lichen Sclerosus

Sallie M. Neill

HISTORICAL BACKGROUND

Lichen sclerosus (LS) is a chronic skin condition, which was first recognized as a possible variant of lichen planus by Hallopeau and Darier in 1887[1]. It can occur at any site, but has a predilection for the genital area, particularly in women. Coincidentally, in 1885, Breisky reported the same condition in the vulva, but called it kraurosis vulvae. This led to the misunderstanding that vulvar lichen sclerosus and kraurosis vulvae were two separate conditions[2]. The nomenclature was further complicated for many years by the additional term, leukoplakic vulvitis[3] and vulvar dystrophy. The International Society for the Study of Vulvovaginal Diseases (ISSVD), together with the International Society of Gynecological Pathologists (ISGYP), has recommended changes in the terminology of vulvar disorders (*see Chapter 12*). As a result, the terms vulvar dystrophy, leukoplakic vulvitis, and kraurosis vulvae have been abandoned, and lichen sclerosus et atrophicus has been abbreviated to lichen sclerosus.

INCIDENCE

The incidence of LS is unknown, but the prevalence has been suggested as between one in 300 and one in 1000 of the population[4]. There are two ages at which the disease is most likely to present – prepuberty and peri- or postmenopause. However, asymptomatic disease is sometimes found coincidentally in women of childbearing age at routine examination and cervical screening.

ETIOLOGY

The etiology is uncertain. In some instances, LS may be familial, affecting siblings and their parents in successive generations[5]. There have been conflicting reports of an association with some types of human leukocyte antigen (HLA)[6]. A possible association with autoimmune disease was first recognized when raised titers of antibodies to thyroid cytoplasm and gastric parietal cells were found in patients with lichen sclerosus[7]. Further reports, supporting an autoimmune basis, have described patients with LS and at least one other autoimmune disease, including vitiligo, lichen planus, morphea, bullous pemphigoid, and thyroid disease[8]. Other immunologic evidence includes fibrin and immunoglobulin deposited along the basement membrane of involved skin[9], and increased numbers of epidermal Langerhans' cells[10].

SYMPTOMS

The major symptom of LS is intense pruritus, so severe that it interferes with sleep. In some cases, however, the patient may be unaware of the disease for years. Pain is an unusual feature, but does occur with deep excoriations and erosions, particularly if there is secondary bacterial infection and cellulitis. Dyspareunia may be a presenting symptom in patients with introital narrowing and tearing at the posterior labial commissure (**16.1**). In children with perianal involvement, painful fissuring of the skin occurs with defecation and the child may then present with constipation.

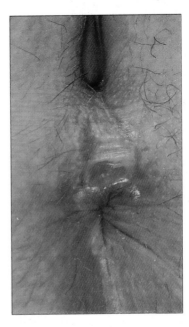

16.1 Lichen sclerosus, affecting the posterior labial commissure, with involvement of the perianal skin and fissuring.

CLINICAL SIGNS

The initial cutaneous signs are usually of pallor, excoriations, and lichenification (**16.2**), with edema and shrinkage of the labia minora (**16.3**). The skin gradually begins to lose its pigmentation and acquires a thinned texture with characteristic 'cigarette paper' wrinkling (**16.4**). There may be purpura and extensive ecchymoses (**16.5**), which occasionally have been mistaken for signs of child abuse. Blistering may be seen, but it is an unusual feature (**16.6**). Eventually, there is architectural distortion with burying of the clitoris under the clitoral hood, resorption of the labia minora, and narrowing of the introitus (**16.7**). There may be a total loss of all the characteristic an-atomic features (**16.8**). Lesions of LS often extend around the perianal area, forming a figure-of-eight configuration (**16.9**), or into the genitocrural folds (**16.10**). The skin in some cases has a warty appearance due to marked hyperkeratosis (**16.11**). Lichen sclerosus does not seem to occur on the non-corn-ified stratified squamous epithelium (i.e. mucosal surfaces), and thus the vagina is spared. There are anecdotal reports of oral involvement, but many of these are probably of lichen planus (LP) (**16.12**). Extragenital involvement occurs in less than a third of patients (**16.13**). There is also an increased incidence of morphea and LP occurring at extra-genital sites in patients with vulvar LS. Postinflam-matory hyperpigmentation is uncommon.

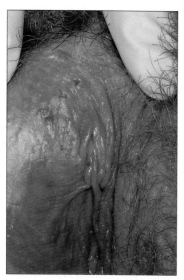

16.2 Lichen sclerosus. Excoriations on a background of lichen sclerosus. There is partial fusion of the anterior labia minora.

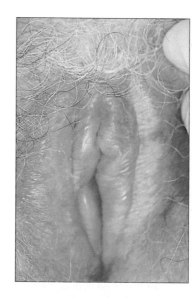

16.3 Lichen sclerosus. There is marked edema of the labia minora and clitoral hood. The skin of the interlabial sulci is white, shiny, and atrophic.

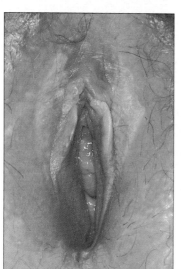

16.4 Lichen sclerosus. Cutaneous atrophy due to lichen sclerosus. The epithelium in the interlabial sulci shows the 'cigarette paper' wrinkling which is characteristic of cutaneous atrophy.

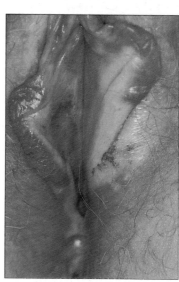

16.5 Lichen sclerosus. There is some asymmetry with more pallor on the left but there is purpura on both sides.

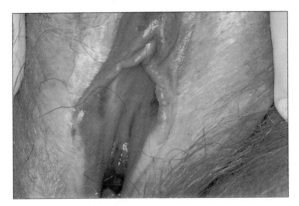

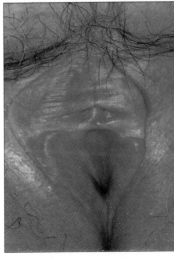

16.7 Lichen sclerosus. There is fusion anteriorly, with burying of the clitoris. The labia minora are merging into the surrounding epithelium and there is marked narrowing of the introitus.

16.6 Lichen sclerosus. The clitoral hood is swollen and small blisters can be seen on the edge of the left labium minorus.

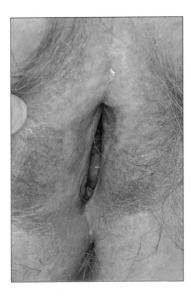

16.8 Lichen sclerosus. The vulva has become featureless with loss of the labia minora, clitoris, and clitoral hood. The introitus is only slightly narrowed.

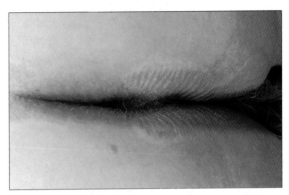

16.9 Lichen sclerosus. Lateral view of perianal area showing lichen sclerosus in a 'figure-of-eight' pattern.

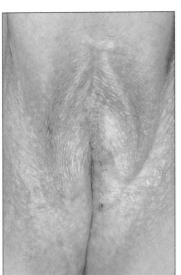

16.10 Lichen sclerosus. This is seen here extending laterally into the genitocrural folds.

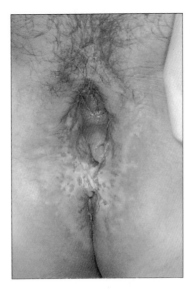

16.11 Lichen sclerosus. The skin across the posterior labial commissure is hyperkeratotic with multiple small erosions.

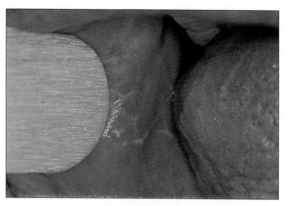

16.12 Lichen planus of the buccal mucosa showing white striae in a reticulate pattern.

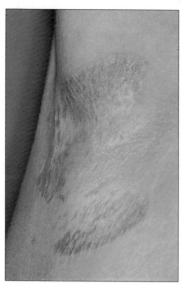

16.13 Extra-genital lichen sclerosus affecting the axilla.

NATURAL HISTORY

There is great variation in the both the area of skin involved and the architectural distortion associated with this condition. Some women have only minimal changes (**16.14**), while in other cases all structure is lost with almost total closure of the introital opening. It was originally believed that childhood LS (**16.15**) went into remission spontaneously with the onset of puberty, but this is no longer believed to be the case. Many patients continue to have the disease, though they may become less symptomatic[11]. It is also inter-esting that many patients improve with pregnancy, but relapse in the puerperium.

About 6% or less of patients with LS develop squamous cell carcinoma. However, LS has been found in about 60% of vulvectomy specimens with squamous cell carcinoma[4,12]. Thus, there would seem to be an important association between LS and squamous cell carcinoma, even though malignancy is a rare complication.

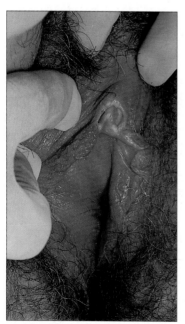

16.14 Localized lichen sclerosus. The area involved may be very limited, as in this patient who has disease localized to the clitoris only.

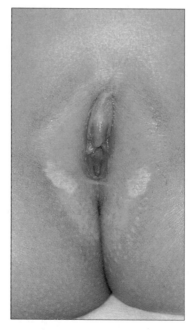

16.15 Child-hood lichen sclerosus. There is generalized pallor of the vulvar skin with two symmetrically arranged plaques of LS either side posteriorly. The clitoral area is also involved.

HISTOLOGY

The typical histology is a thinned, effaced epidermis, with or without overlying hyperkeratosis. In the reticular dermis, immediately underneath the epidermis, there is a band of homogenized collagen. An associated lymphocytic infiltrate may be seen just beneath this abnormal dermis (**16.16**). Occasionally, this lymphocytic infiltrate is high in the dermis, occurring along the dermoepidermal junction with areas of basal cell liquefaction very similar to the changes seen in LP[13]. In some cases, the epidermis is acanthotic showing squamous cell hyperplasia (**16.17**). It has been suggested that this type of LS is more frequently associated with squamous cell carcinoma[14,15].

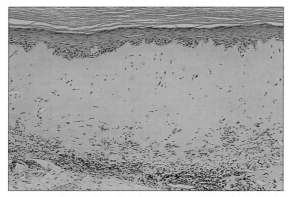

16.16 Lichen sclerosus showing epidermal atrophy with overlying hyperkeratosis, and upper dermal hyalinization with cellular infiltrate underneath. (Hematoxylin & eosin stain x 40.)

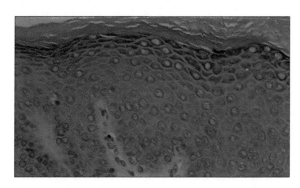

16.17 Squamous cell hyperplasia. Lichen sclerosus with squamous cell hyperplasia. (Hematoxylin & eosin stain x 400.)

MANAGEMENT

MEDICAL TREATMENT

The treatment of choice is a potent topical corticosteroid, such as clobetasol propionate 0.05%[16]. This is applied to the affected skin once daily, usually at night, until there is an improvement, after which the frequency can gradually be reduced. Patient information and instruction leaflets are invaluable. It is important to monitor the amount of topical steroid used. A 30g tube should last three months, but considerably less is required once the disease is under control.

Despite the high incidence of LS at the time of the menopause and the apparent improvement in pregnancy, both systemic and topical exogenous estrogens are ineffective in the treatment of LS. Similarly, topical testosterone acts mainly as an emollient and is no longer a recognized treatment. There are anecdotal reports of systemic and topical synthetic retinoids being used to treat vulvar LS, but these should probably be reserved for cases that fail to respond to topical corticosteroids. A soap substitute, such as aqueous cream, is a useful adjunct to treatment. (*See also Patient Information Sheets*, pp.182-183.)

SURGERY

A vulvectomy should never be performed for treatment of this disorder, except when it has been complicated by the development of squamous cell carcinoma (**16.18**). Otherwise, surgical intervention

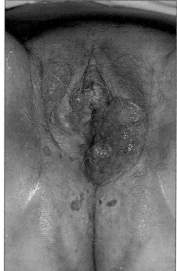

16.18 Squamous cell carcinoma. A large fungating squamous cell carcinoma arising on a background of lichen sclerosus which had not previously been diagnosed or treated.

should only be considered when there has been such extensive labial fusion that it is necessary to reconstruct an introitus (**16.19**). A vulvoperineoplasty is then recommended which uses part of the posterior vaginal wall in the reconstruction[17].

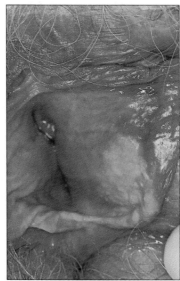

16.20 Vulvar intraepithelial neoplasia (VIN). Biopsy of these white plaques showed full-thickness atypia, consistent with the diagnosis of VIN 3.

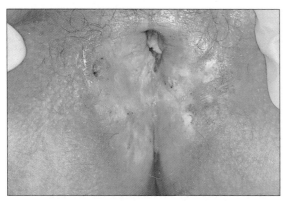

16.19 Severe introital narrowing which interfered with micturition. In younger patients, this degree of narrowing would affect sexual function.

DIFFERENTIAL DIAGNOSIS

Leukoplakia literally means 'white plaque' and is not a diagnosis in itself. It should therefore be used only as a descriptive term. Lichen sclerosus is only one of a number of conditions which result in the formation of white plaques associated with pallor, scarring, and atrophy. These changes can also represent the end-stage appearance for many dermatoses (*see Chapter 13 and Appendix A*).

Human papillomavirus infection, with or without vulvar intraepithelial neoplasia (**16.20**), may be another cause of white plaques, but atrophy and scarring would be unusual features. A skin biopsy is always important to establish a definite diagnosis, and direct and indirect immunofluorescence studies should be done if there are diagnostic difficulties.

REFERENCES
1 Hallopeau, H. Lichen plan sclereux. *Ann. Dermatol. Syph.* 1889; 10: 447–449.
2 Breisky, D. Uber kraurosis vulvae. *Z. Heilkd.* 1885; 6: 69–80.
3 Berkeley, C. M. B. and Bonney, V. M. S. Leukoplakic vulvitis and its relation to kraurosis vulvae and carcinoma vulvae. *Proc. Roy. Soc. Med. (Obstet. Gynaecol. Section)* 1909; 3: 29–51.
4 Wallace, H. J. Lichen sclerosus et atrophicus. *Trans. St. John's Dermatol. Soc.* 1971; 57: 9–30.
5 Ridley, C. M. General dermatologic conditions and dermatoses of the vulva. In: Ridley, C. M. (ed.) *The Vulva.* Edinburgh: Churchill Livingstone, 1988: pp.138– 211.
6 Purcell, K. G., Spencer, L. V., Simpson, P. M., *et al.* HLA antigens in lichen sclerosus et atrophicus. *Arch. Dermatol.* 1990; 126: 1043–1045.
7 Goolamali, S. K., Barnes, E. W., Irvine, W. J., *et al.* Organ specific antibodies in patients with lichen sclerosus. *Br. Med. J.* 1974; iv: 78–79.
8 Harrington, C. I. and Dunsmore, I. R. An investigation into the incidence of autoimmune disorders in patients with lichen sclerosus et atrophicus. *Br. J. Dermatol.* 1981; 104: 563–566.
9 Dickie, R. J., Horne, C. H. W., and Sutherland, H. W. Direct evidence of localized immunologic damage in lichen sclerosus et atrophicus. *J. Clin. Pathol.* 1982; 35: 1395–1399.
10 Carli, P., Cattaneo, A., Pimpenelli N., *et al.* Immunohistochemical evidence of skin immune system involvement in vulvar lichen sclerosus et atrophicus. *Dermatologica* 1991; 182: 18–22.
11 Ridley, C. M. Genital lichen sclerosus (lichen sclerosus et atrophicus) in childhood and adolescence. *J. Roy. Soc. Med.* 1993; 86: 69–75.
12 Leibowitch, M., Neill, S., Pelisse, M., *et al.* The epithelial changes associated with squamous cell carcinoma of the vulva: a review of the clinical, histologic and viral findings in 78 women. *Br. J. Obstet. Gynaecol.* 1990; 97: 1135–1139.
13 Hewitt, J. Histologic criteria for lichen sclerosus of the vulva. *J. Reprod. Med.* 1986; 31: 781–787.
14 Rodke, G., Friedrich, E. G., and Wilkinson, E. J. Malignant potential of mixed vulvar dystrophy (lichen sclerosus associated with squamous cell hyperplasia). *J. Reprod. Med.* 1988; 33: 545–550.
15 Hart, W. R., Norris, J., and Helwig, E. B. Relation of lichen sclerosus et atrophicus of the vulva to development of carcinoma. *Obstet. Gynecol.* 1975; 45: 369–377.
16 Dalziel, K., Millard, P. R., and Wojnarowska, F. The treatment of vulvar lichen sclerosus with a very potent topical corticosteroid (clobetasol propionate 0.05%) cream. *Br. J. Dermatol.* 1991; 124: 461–464.
17 Paniel, B. J., Truc, J. B, de Margerie, V., *et al.* La vulvo-perineoplastie. *J. Gynecol. Obstet. Biol. Reprod.* 1984; 1: 91–99.

17.
Erosive Vulvovaginitis

Pauline Marren & Fenella Wojnarowska

INTRODUCTION

Erosion is the loss of epidermis, and can occur with a variety of inflammatory, bullous, infective, and neoplastic processes. Ulcers are deeper than erosions, though there is overlap in the differential diagnoses (*see Appendix A*). The diagnosis is often difficult, as lesions may be generalized, limited to mucosae, or localized to one region. Examination of the vulvovaginal area must be combined with a thorough examination of the skin, all mucosal sites, hair, and nails, so that the diagnosis is based on a complete clinical picture.

Erosions may form after loss of a fragile blister roof (pemphigus), or from intertriginous rubbing and breakage of tense, otherwise resilient, blisters (bullous pemphigoid). Excoriations are erosions caused by the patient's scratching, and are a secondary feature of pruritic vulvar dermatoses. In the past 20 years, much progress has been made in the differential diagnosis of 'erosive vaginitis', but some cases still cannot be classified clinically or histologically. These idiopathic forms may represent vulvovaginal diseases that have not yet been characterized.

EROSIVE LICHEN PLANUS

Mucocutaneous lichen planus (LP) is a relatively common condition characterized by itchy, violaceous, flat-topped papules on cutaneous sites (**17.1**),

and less clearly defined reticulated, white and violaceous papules or plaques on oral and vulvar skin (**17.2**, **17.3**). Cutaneous and oral involvement is common, either separately or in combination, but the frequency of benign vulvar involvement is unknown[1].

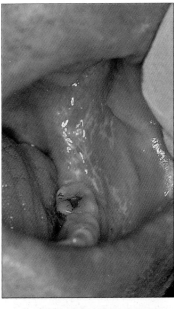

17.2 Lichen planus of the mouth with reticulated white plaques.

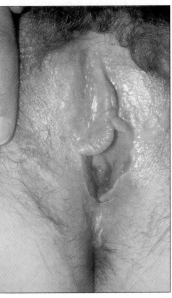

17.3 Lichen planus of the vulva with violaceous border.

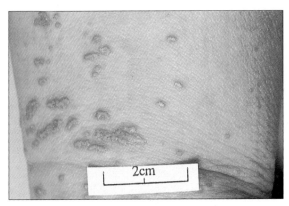

17.1 Lichen planus with typical violaceous papules on skin surfaces.

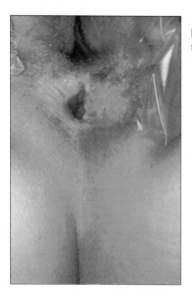

17.4 Erosive lichen planus of the vulva.

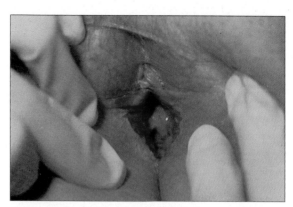

17.5 Erosive lichen planus of the vulva.

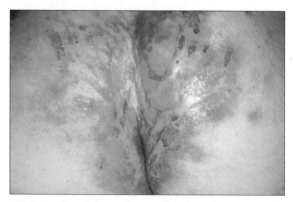

17.6 Erosive lichen planus of the buttocks and perianal skin.

Erosive LP (vulvo-vaginal-gingival syndrome) was first described as a distinct entity in 1982[2], and is a well-defined, though uncommon, subgroup. The characteristic feature is severe and extensive erosion and ulceration at affected sites with prolonged clinical courses which are a difficult therapeutic challenge. It is generally believed that patients with erosive LP will develop erosive lesions at vulvar, vaginal, and gingival sites, at some stage in the course of their disease, though all three sites may not be concurrently affected. The site of the presenting symptom determines the referring physician: gynecologist, dermatologist, or oral specialist. About 20–30% of these patients also have evidence of cutaneous or scalp involvement. Lichen planus is uncommon in children[3], and the erosive form has only been described in adults.

Vulvar symptoms are often severe and unremitting. Patients complain of pain, burning, dyspareunia, and postcoital bleeding. Frank erosion may vary in degree and extent, but can encircle the entire introitus (**17.4, 17.5**). Eroded areas may be surrounded by a reticulated white border. Vulvar adhesions and labial atrophy with fusion and clitoral burial, together with loss of tissue mass, are common. The keratinized skin in the perineal and perianal area tends to show the classic violaceous papules and plaques of LP, which can be helpful in diagnosis (**17.6**).

One-half to two-thirds of patients with erosive LP have vaginal involvement during the course of the disease[4,5]. Episodes of vaginitis do not necessarily correlate in time with the appearance of vulvitis, and symptoms vary in severity, with periods of regression. The insertion of a vaginal speculum can be exceedingly painful, and sometimes impossible, because of vaginal adhesions. There may be either a generalized vaginitis that is friable,

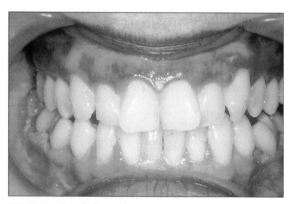

17.7 Erosive lichen planus of the mouth.

desquamative, and hemorrhagic, or less extensive erosions with an overlying white lacy network. The cervix can be friable and desquamative, and may be obscured from view by stenosis of the upper vagina.

Although tender, friable gingivitis is an uncommon presenting complaint, it will develop at some time during the course of the disease in two-thirds to three-quarters of patients. Gingival erosion and desquamation can be localized or generalized, and erosions are sometimes surrounded by a white rim (**17.7**).

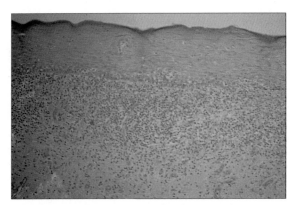

17.8 Lichen planus. Biopsy of oral mucosa showing features of lichen planus.

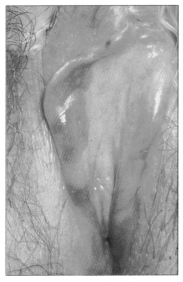

17.9 'Glazed erythema' of the vulva.

DIAGNOSIS

Biopsies should be taken from the border of an eroded area for histopathology and direct immuno-fluorescence. An experienced dermatopathologist can be extremely helpful in the interpretation of mucosal sections. The typical histologic features of LP are a subepidermal band-like inflammatory in-filtrate and some basal cell degenerative changes, with or without cytoid bodies (**17.8**). Direct immuno-fluorescence (IF) with colloid bodies may support the diagnosis, while the typical clinical morphology and distribution of LP lesions can support the diagnosis when histology is equivocal.

Differential Diagnosis

Autoimmune blistering diseases can also present with an erosive gingivitis, vulvitis, cervicitis, or vagin-itis. Of these, cicatricial pemphigoid is clinically most like erosive LP (*see below*). A general physical exam-ination is essential to exclude evidence of either dis-ease at other sites. Direct and indirect IF studies are helpful in differentiating these disorders. Vulvitis cir-cumscripta plasmacellularis (plasma cell vulvitis, Zoon's erythroplasia) can present with well-demarc-ated erosions on the labia minora, but oral and vag-inal involvement are not characteristic[6] and histology tends to be more specific. Erosive vaginitis with ad-hesions has been described in many patients with graft-versus-host-disease (GVHD), a condition which is also associated with lichenoid cutaneous erupt-ions. Biopsy is recommended to differentiate between the variety of possible diagnostic considerations[7] (*see Appendix A*).

Finally, the authors recognize a superficially erod-ed shiny glazed vulvitis with non-specific inflammat-ory histology, which so far has defied diagnostic categorization, and which we have descriptively named 'glazed erythema' (**17.9**). This characteristically runs a protracted course and can be very symptomatic, but has no oral or vaginal involvement.

MANAGEMENT

Erosive LP is chronic and recalcitrant. These patients probably also have an increased risk of developing squamous cell carcinoma. This supposition is based on the well-documented risk of squamous cell carcin-oma in erosive oral and penile LP[8,9]. It would be logic-al to assume that patients with vulvovaginal lesions share a similar risk. Certainly, patients should be carefully monitored throughout the course of their disease. There is no ideal treatment for this disorder, but there are several possible therapies which have proved helpful in some cases. (*See also Patient In-formation Sheets*, pp.180–181.)

Topical Treatment

Aqueous cream emollients are soothing, and the dis-comfort of towel drying can be avoided by using a hand-held hairdryer at low temperature. Some patients may find that potent topical steroids (e.g. clobetas-ol propionate 0.05%) are very helpful. Rectal prepar-ations such as hydrocortisone acetate 10% and prednisolone suppositories are useful for vaginal lesions. In one series, only about 25% of patients showed satisfactory improvement with topical pre-parations[3]. Although topical cyclosporin 'swish' therapy has been helpful in treating erosive oral LP[10–12], it has been disappointing in vulvovaginal lesions[13]. Treatment is very costly and could theoretically increase the risk of malignancy. Topically applied tretinoin and isotretinoin are only beneficial for non-erosive oral lesions[14]. Their usefulness is limited by local irritation in the vulvovaginal area.

Systemic Treatment

Oral steroid therapy (at least 0.5mg/kg/day) is helpful in about 50% of patients treated[3], but erosions recur on tapering. Intralesional steroid injections can be helpful in some cases. There are several reports of the use of systemic retinoids (acitretin, etretinate, isotretinoin) in mucosal LP[15–18], but these drugs are potent teratogens with prolonged half-lives, which seriously limits their use in women of childbearing age. Clearly, the efficacy of systemic retinoids for treating erosive LP at all sites will require further evaluation and the support of adequate clinical trials. In addition to teratogenicity, retinoids often cause skin fragility, hair loss, muscle cramps, headaches, increased levels of serum triglycerides, and rarely, acute severe hepatitis.

Oral griseofulvin has been described as a useful therapy for severe LP[19–21], but not for erosive vulvar disease. There have also been anecdotal reports of the beneficial use of dapsone in severe erosive oral and acral forms of the disease[22,23], and hydroxychloroquine sulfate has been helpful in treating erosive LP[24]. There is no ideal treatment for erosive vulvar LP.

Many systemic treatments are limited by their side-effects and/or are unsuitable as maintenance therapy.

Surgery

Juxtaposed erosive surfaces tend to form adhesions or synechiae. This is the most likely reason for recurrence in patients who have undergone surgical division of adhesions. Laser ablation is not effective[4], and split-skin grafting has not yet been reported. In severe cases, in which urethral or menstrual function are compromised, blunt dissection of mucosal adhesions can be performed. Potent topical steroids should be applied postoperatively with vaginal dilators to minimize inflammation during healing. When only the anterior vagina is involved, function can often be restored by surgery, and maintained afterwards with topical steroids.

BULLOUS DISEASES

The autoimmune blistering diseases affect skin and mucous membrane sites, including the vulvovaginal area (**Table 17.1**). Autoantibodies directed against normal components of the epithelium and basement membrane zone (BMZ) mediate these diseases. The target antigens are those involved in the adhesion of epithelial cells to each other, or to the underlying

Disease	Patients	Distribution	Mucosal lesions	Vulvovaginal	Lesions	Scarring	Treatment	Prognosis
Pemphigus vulgaris	Adults	Generalized	Always major	+++ (80%)	Flaccid blisters, erosions		Steroids, immuno-suppressants	Most remit
Bullous pemphigoid	Elderly (rare in children)	Trunk, limbs, flexures	Common, minor	+ (9%)	Urticated plaques, tense blisters (milia)		Steroids, dapsone, immuno-suppressants	3–4 years
Cicatricial pemphigoid	middle to old age	Infrequent	Major, severe	+++ (53%) scarring	Erosions, blisters, gingivitis, milia	+++	Steroids, dapsone, immuno-suppressants	Chronic
Linear IgA disease (CBDC and adults)	Children and elderly	Perineum, face, trunk, limbs	Majority (few severe)	++ (60%) children > adults	Urticated plaques, anular lesions, tense blisters	+ (mucosae, rare)	Dapsone, sulfon-amides	3–4 years (few persist)
Epidermolysis bullosa acquisita	Adults (few children)	Generalized, variable	Some (few severe)	++ (60%)	Urticated plaques, tense blisters, milia	++	Steroids, dapsone, immuno-suppressants	Persists

Table 17.1 Clinical Features of the Autoimmune Bullous Diseases.

| Disease | Immuno-fluorescence | Autoantibodies | | | |
		Isotype	Binding to split skin	Target antigens	Antigen weight (kDa)
Pemphigus vulgaris	Intraepidermal	IgG		PV antigen	140
Bullous pemphigoid	Linear BMZ	IgG, few IgA	Epidermal	BPA-1 BPA-2	220 180
Cicatricial pemphigoid	Linear BMZ	IgG, IgA	Epidermal Dermal	BPA-1 BPA-2 Epiligrin/nicein Others	220 180 600
Linear IgA disease (CBDC and adults)	Linear BMZ	IgA	Epidermal (majority) Dermal (minority)	? (Few BPA-1 and BPA-2)	285, 97 (Few 180, 220)
Epidermolysis bullosa acquisita	Linear BMZ	IgG	Dermal	Collagen VII (anchoring fibril)	290

Table 17.2 Immunopathology of the Autoimmune Bullous Diseases.

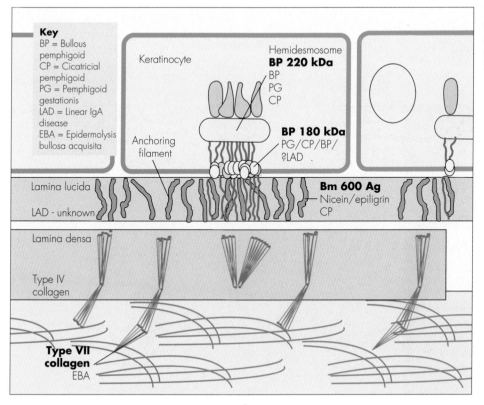

17.10 Localization of target antigens in the autoimmune bullous diseases.

stroma (**Table 17.2**). Their ultrastructural localization is shown in **17.10**.

At cutaneous sites, this antigen–antibody interaction provokes a characteristic blister, although erosion is more common at mucosal sites, where it can be clinically indistinguishable from erosion due to other causes. However, diagnosis is not usually a problem, as autoimmune blistering diseases usually affect both skin and mucosal sites. If, as occasionally occurs, only the mucosae are affected, then diagnosis may be difficult; appropriate laboratory investigations are essential for diagnostic accuracy in cases where a blistering disease is a possibility.

PEMPHIGUS VULGARIS

Pemphigus vulgaris is the most common type of pemphigus, affecting about 80% of pemphigus patients. The peak incidence of occurrence is between the fourth and sixth decade. Cutaneous blisters are flaccid and fragile, rupturing to produce raw, denuded areas (**17.11**). Extensive involvement can be life-threatening. Mucous membrane involvement affects 85–90% of patients (**17.12**). Other mucosal sites include the nose, conjunctiva, larynx, pharynx, esophagus, urethra, and cervix. Vulvovaginal involvement is common[25]; lesions are erosive, painful and can be extensive (**17.13**).

Histology of a fresh intact cutaneous blister will show the characteristic intraepidermal blister containing rounded acantholytic cells. Immunofluorescence studies are vital in suspected cases and should be repeated if necessary. Punch biopsies are ideal for this purpose and can be performed under local anesthetic. Direct IF from perilesional skin or mucosa as well as an uninvolved site, and indirect IF of serum, should be performed. IgG deposition and binding of patient's sera to the epidermal cell surface occurs in over 90% of patients with pemphigus vulgaris (**17.14**).

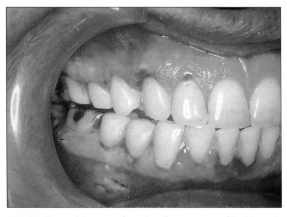

17.12 Pemphigus vulgaris affecting gingival surfaces.

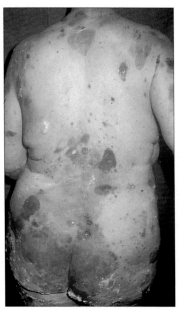

17.11 Pemphigus vulgaris. Extensive pemphigus vulgaris affecting cutaneous sites.

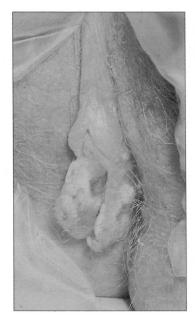

17.13 Pemphigus vulgaris with prominent vulvar erosions.

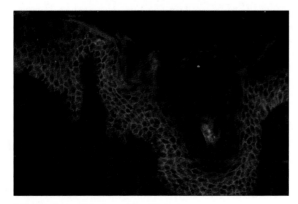

17.14 Pemphigus vulgaris. Indirect immuno-fluorescence with IgG deposition on the surface of epidermal cells.

BULLOUS PEMPHIGOID

Bullous pemphigoid (BP) is the commonest of all blistering diseases. Generally, it affects the elderly, though cases have been reported in childhood. Skin involvement may be localized or extensive; blisters are usually tense and may arise on normal or urticated skin (**17.15**). Two years is the average time

until remission occurs. Mucosal sites are involved in over 50% of cases[25]. Labial erosions cause pain, itch, and dysuria (**17.16**). Localized vulvar pemphigoid has been described in children[26,27]. Mucosal sites affected include the vagina, oral and nasal mucosa, the pharynx, conjunctiva, esophagus, and anus. Lesions heal without scarring, so examination can be normal when the disease is in control or in remission.

The histology of a fresh intact cutaneous blister shows a subepidermal split at the dermoepidermal junction, with a mixed dermal inflammatory infiltrate consisting of numerous eosinophils. Direct and indirect IF studies can aid diagnosis, as shown in **Table 17.2** and in **17.17**. Antibodies to BP generally bind to

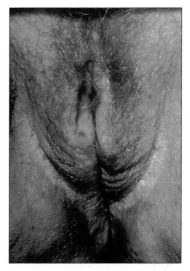

17.16 Bullous pemphigoid of the vulva with erosions.

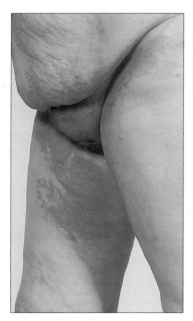

17.15 Bullous pemphigoid. Urticated plaque in the pre-blistering phase of bullous pemphigoid.

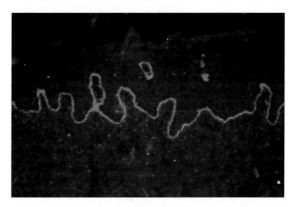

17.17 Bullous pemphigoid. Linear dermoepidermal band on indirect immunofluorescence using vaginal mucosa.

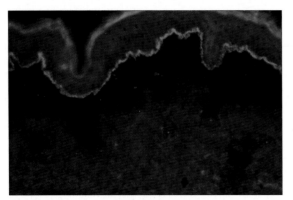

17.18 Bullous pemphigoid. Indirect immuno-fluorescence on bullous pemphigoid serum showing binding to the roof on salt-split skin.

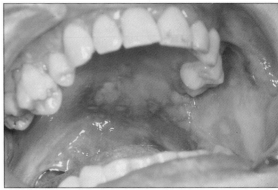

17.19 Cicatricial pemphigoid of the mouth with erosions.

the roof of a split skin preparation (**17.18**), differentiating BP from epidermolysis bullosa acquisita in which antibodies bind to the base.

CICATRICIAL PEMPHIGOID

Cicatricial pemphigoid (CP), a scarring bullous disease, predominantly affects mucosal surfaces. Cutaneous lesions occur in only 10–25% of cases, and vulvar scarring is often indistinguishable from that of erosive LP. CP usually affects the middle-aged and elderly. Oral lesions include blisters, erosions, and/or gingivitis (**17.19**); other affected sites are the conjunctiva (**17.20**), nasal mucosa, larynx, pharynx, and esophagus. Scarring and morbidity can be significant in the eye (blindness), the larynx (stridor), and the esophagus (dysphagia).

Erosions can develop on the labia, urethra, vagina, rectum, or perianal skin (**17.21**). Patients complain of soreness, pain, itch, and urethral symptoms. Scarring with labial fusion is common, with or without clitoral burial, and vaginal introital stenosis may make intercourse difficult or impossible. Urethral stenosis may also require dilatation. The disease is typically difficult to treat and unfortunately there is no tendency towards spontaneous resolution.

CP is essentially a clinical diagnosis; biopsy of a fresh intact cutaneous blister will show a subepidermal split and there may be scarring in the dermis. Direct IF is often negative in CP, though some authors have found that biopsies from buccal and conjunctival mucosae give the best positive yield. Multiple biopsies should ideally be taken to increase the likelihood of accurate diagnosis. The use of split-skin as a substrate undoubtedly gives the highest positive yield with binding of IgG or IgA autoantibodies to the

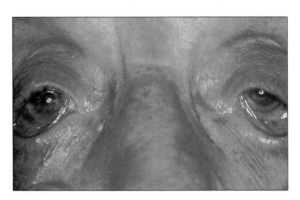

17.20 Cicatricial pemphigoid of the eyes with conjunctival scarring.

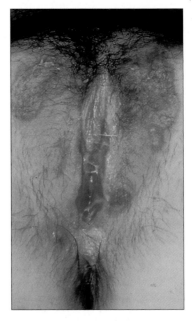

17.21 Cicatricial pemphigoid with severe vulvar erosion.

roof in most cases of CP, though some do bind to the floor[28]. Despite differences in the clinical expression of the two diseases, the target antigens are shared with BP.

EPIDERMOLYSIS BULLOSA ACQUISITA

Epidermolysis bullosa acquisita (EBA) is an uncommon blistering disease. It is characterized by skin fragility and erosion with a tendency to heal with scarring[29], and thus may be indistinguishable from bullous and cicatricial pemphigoid (**17.22**). Mucous membrane involvement affecting the mouth, eyes, esophagus, and larynx is common, and vulvar scarring may lead to introital stenosis and functional disability.

The histology of EBA is similar to that of pemphigoid. Direct IF shows IgG deposited in a linear band at the dermoepidermal junction, while indirect IF is positive in many patients. The use of salt split-skin improves the diagnostic yield, and the dermal binding of IgG distinguishes EBA from BP[30].

sexual abuse. Adults can present with widespread blistering on cutaneous and mucosal sites, including the mouth, eyes, nasopharynx, larynx, esophagus, and trachea.

Histology of a fresh intact blister shows that the blister is subepidermal (**17.24**). Direct IF demonstrates a linear band of IgA at the BMZ in all cases. Indirect IF is positive for IgA autoantibodies in most children and some adults.

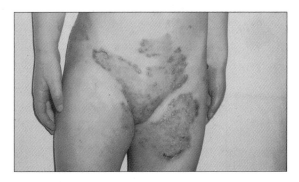

17.23 Linear IgA disease. Typical lesions are shown in linear IgA disease (chronic bullous disease of childhood).

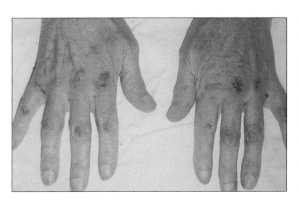

17.22 Epidermolysis bullosa acquisita of the hands with fragility and erosions.

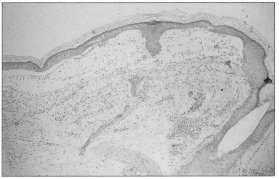

17.24 Linear IgA disease. Histology of linear IgA disease with subepidermal blistering.

LINEAR IgA DISEASE

This uncommon blistering disease has been described in both adults and children (formerly called chronic bullous disease of childhood)[31]. The most characteristic lesion of linear IgA disease is the annular polycyclic or gyrate lesion with a peripheral ring of blistering. Children present with blisters, some of which are hemorrhagic, most commonly on or near the genital or perioral areas[25]. With time, blisters become more generalized, and mucosal involvement with scarring can be a feature (**17.23**). Some children have been mistakenly diagnosed as being victims of

MANAGEMENT

Potent topical corticosteroid preparations and treatment of secondary infection are the mainstays of local therapy for autoimmune bullous diseases. Systemic therapy may be necessary in generalized or extensive disease and is outlined in **Table 17.1**. The current armamentarium includes systemic corticosteroids, dapsone, sulfonamides, minocycline (sometimes with nicotinamide), and azathioprine. Each case must be carefully and individually assessed in the light of the patient's general health and her ability to tolerate the different treatment regimes. Multiple drug combinations are sometimes required for severe cases, and all patients need to be closely monitored for hematologic and hepatic side effects. Surgical intervention may be necessary when there is functional impairment of the vulva, esophagus, or larynx.

GENETICALLY DETERMINED BULLOUS DISEASES

Epidermolysis Bullosa Dystrophica

Epidermolysis bullosa dystrophica is a rare blistering disease, which can be inherited as an autosomal-dominant or autosomal-recessive trait. The genetic cause is a mutation of collagen VII, which is the major component of the anchoring fibrils (*see* **17.10**). This results in faulty adhesion of the epidermis to the dermis, producing repeated blistering with dystrophic scarring and deformity. Most patients present in infancy. The involvement of mucous membranes is a constant feature of the severe form of recessive epidermolysis bullosa dystrophica. Scarring leads to a variety of complications including:

• Microstomia;
• Limited mobility of the tongue;
• Gingival retraction and dental decay;
• Esophageal stenosis;
• Corneal scarring;
• Anal stenosis.

Blistering, erosion, and scarring of the vulva, introitus, vagina, and perineal and perianal skin have also been reported as leading to vaginal stenosis[32]. The diagnosis is established by electron microscopy, which is used to determine the level of separation in the BMZ, and by immunohistochemical techniques, which are used to demonstrate the absence of collagen VII in the recessive disease. Treatment is mainly supportive.

Hailey–Hailey Disease (Benign Familial Pemphigus)

Patients with autosomal-dominant benign familial pemphigus have recurrent vesicular lesions or crusted erosions in intertriginous areas, including the axillary, inframammary and perineal areas, and the groin[33]. The morphology varies from expanding plaques with scaly borders simulating fungal infections, to crusted erosions and vesicopustules. Hypertrophic perineal involvement may be mistaken for chronic *Candida* infection or malignancy. Cases have been reported confined to the vulva[34]. Intact blisters are uncommon (**17.25**). Diagnosis is established histologically in cases when the typical suprabasal acantholysis can be identified. Topical steroids and the treatment of secondary infection can provide considerable amelioration, but flares and remissions are typical.

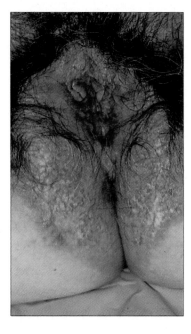

17.25 Hailey–Hailey disease of the vulva.

CONCLUSION

Erosive conditions of the vulva are a misery to patients and taxing to physicians. Diagnosis is often difficult, prognosis is usually uncertain, and treatment is often disappointing. The mainstay of diagnosis remains the clinical history and examination.

REFERENCES

1 Boyd, A. S. and Nelder, K. H. Lichen planus. *J. Am. Acad. Dermatol.* 1991; **25**: 593–619.

2 Pelisse, M., Leibowitch, M., Sedel, D., *et al.* Un nouveau syndrome vulvo-vagino-gingival. Lichen plan erosif plurimuqueux. *Ann. Dermatol. Venereol. (Paris)* 1982; **109**: 797–798.

3 Kanwar, A. J., Handa, S., Ghosh, S., *et al.* Lichen planus in childhood: a report in 17 patients. *Pediatr. Dermatol.* 1991; **8**: 288–291.

4 Pelisse, M. The vulvo-vaginal-gingival syndrome. A new form of erosive lichen planus. *Int. J. Dermatol.* 1989; **28**: 381–384.

5 Ridley, C. M. Chronic erosive vulval disease. *Clin. Experim. Dermatol.* 1990; **15**: 245–252.

6 Davis, J., Shapiro, L., and Baral, J. Vulvitis circumscripta plasmacellularis. *J. Am. Acad. Dermatol.* 1983; **8**: 413–416.

7 Edwards, L. Desquamative vulvitis. *Dermatol. Clin.* (vulvar diseases) 1992; **10**: 325–337.

8 Harland, C. C., Fallowfield, M. E., Marsden, R. A., *et al.* Squamous carcinoma complicating lichen planus of the lip. *Br. J. Dermatol.* 1991; **125**(suppl.38): 96–97.

9 Marder, M. Z. and Deesen, K. C. Transformation of oral lichen planus to squamous cell carcinoma: a literature review and report of a case. *J. Am. Dent. Assoc.* 1982; **105**: 55–60.

10 Eisen, D., Griffiths, C. E. M., Ellis, C. N., *et al.* Cyclosporin wash for oral lichen planus (letter). *Lancet* 1990; **335**: 535–536.

11 Balato, N., De Rosa, S., Bordone, F., *et al.* Dermatological application of cyclosporin. *Arch. Dermatol.* 1989; **125**: 430–431.

12 Frances, C., Boisnic, S., Etienne, S., *et al.* Effect of the local application of cyclosporin A on chronic erosive lichen planus of the oral cavity. *Dermatologica* 1988; **177**: 194–195.

13 Pelisse, M. Presented at the 11th International Congress of the International Society for the Study of Vulvar Disease. Oxford, England, September 1991.

14 Giustina, T. A., Stewart, J. C. B., Ellis, C. N., *et al.* Topical application of isotretinoin gel improves oral lichen planus. *Arch. Dermatol.* 1986; **122**: 534–536.

15 Laurberg, G., Geiger, J. M., Hjorth, N., *et al.* Treatment of lichen planus with acitretin. *J. Am. Acad. Dermatol.* 1991; **24**: 434–437.

16 Hersle, K., Mobacken, H., Sloberg, K., *et al.* Severe oral lichen planus: treatment with an aromatic retinoid (etretinate). *Br. J. Dermatol.* 1982; **106**: 77–80.

17 Woo, T. Y. Systemic isotretinoin treatment of oral and cutaneous lichen planus. *Cutis* 1985; **35**(4): 385–393.

18 Staus, M. E. and Bergfeld, W. F. Treatment of oral lichen planus with low-dose isotretinoin. *J. Am. Acad. Dermatol.* 1984: **11**(3): 527–528.

19 Massa, M. C. and Rogers, R. S. Griseofulvin therapy of lichen planus. *Acta Dermato. Venereol. (Stockholm)* 1981; **61**: 547–550.

20 Sehgal, V. N., Abraham, G. J. S., and Malik, G. B. Griseofulvin therapy in lichen planus. *Br. J. Dermatol.* 1972; **87**: 383.

21 Meyrick Thomas, R. H., Munro, D. D., and Robinson, T. W. E. Erosive lichen planus treated with griseofulvin. *Br. J. Dermatol.* 1983; **109**(suppl.24): 97–98.

22 Falk, D. K., Latour, D. L., and King, L. E. Dapsone in the treatment of erosive lichen planus. *J. Am. Acad. Dermatol.* 1985; **12**: 567–570.

23 Beck, H. I. and Brandrup, F. Treatment of erosive lichen planus with dapsone. *Acta Dermato. Venereol. (Stockholm)* 1986; **66**: 366–367.

24 Eisen, D. Hydroxychloroquine sulfate (Plaquenil) improves oral lichen planus. *J. Am. Acad. Dermatol.* 1993; **28**: 609–612.

25 Marren, P., Wojnarowska, F., Venning, V., *et al.* Vulvar involvement in autoimmune bullous diseases. *J. Reprod. Med.* 1993; **38**(2): 101–107.

26 Oranje, A. P. and Van Joost, T. Pemphigoid in children. *Pediatr. Dermatol.* 1989; **6**(4): 267–274.

27 DeCastro, P., Jorizzo, J. L., and Rajaraman, S. Localized vulvar pemphigoid in a child. *Pediatr. Dermatol.* 1985; **2**: 302–307.

28 Allen, J., Schomberg, K., Venning, V. A., *et al.* A comparison of the localization of the antibodies and antigens in cicatricial pemphigoid. *Br. J. Dermatol.* 1992; **127**: 430.

29 Roenigk, H. H. Jr., Ryan, J. G., and Bergfeld, W. F. Epidermolysis bullosa acquisita: report of three cases and review of all published cases. *Arch. Dermatol.* 1971; **103**: 1–10.

30 Yaoita, H., Briggaman, R. A., Lawley, T. J., *et al.* Epidermolysis bullosa acquisita: ultrastructural and immunological studies. *J. Invest. Dermatol.* 1981; **76**: 288–292.

31 Wojnarowska, F., Marsden, R. A., Bhogal, B., *et al.* Chronic bullous disease of childhood, childhood cicatricial pemphigoid and linear IgA disease of adults: a comparative study demonstrating clinical and immunopathological overlap. *J. Am. Acad. Dermatol.* 1988; **19**: 792–805.

32 Shakelford, G., Bauer, E., Graviss, E. R., *et al.* Upper airway and external genital involvement in epidermolysis bullosa dystrophica. *Radiology* 1982; **143**: 429–432.

33 Burge, S. M. Hailey-Hailey disease; the clinical features, response to treatment, and prognosis. *Br. J. Dermatol.* 1992; **126**: 275–282.

34 Thiers, H., Moulin, G., Rochet, Y., *et al.* Maladie de Hailey-Hailey: a localisation vulvaire predominante. Etude génétique et ultrastructurale. *Bulletin Société Française Dermatologie Syphiligraphie* 1968; **75**: 352–355.

18.
Vulvar Manifestations of Systemic Disease

Christine Harrington

INTRODUCTION

Vulvar symptoms usually result from a primary dermatosis, or from a generalized skin disease which involves the vulva. Occasionally, vulvar lesions are manifestations or complications of systemic disease, and, rarely, the vulva may be the site of presentation of a systemic disorder. If systemic disease is suspected, a detailed history should be taken, and the skin and mucous membranes should be thoroughly examined. Vulvar biopsy and appropriate investigations will be needed to confirm the diagnosis and to guide appropriate management.

CHRONIC PRURITUS VULVAE (LICHEN SIMPLEX CHRONICUS)

Persistent scratching of the vulva causes lichenification, usually of the labia majora. The skin may be leathery and thickened (**18.1**), or may become eroded in severe cases (**18.2**). While the underlying cause is being investigated, a moderately potent topical steroid and a systemic antipruritic agent may be used to alleviate the itch[1].

Iron-Deficiency Anemia
Iron-deficiency anemia causes chronic pruritus; occasionally, the itch is localized to the vulva. Causes of iron-deficiency anemia should be considered in the history and examination of a patient with unexplained pruritus vulvae[2]. Possible causes include a poor diet or blood loss from menorrhagia, hemorrhoids, or gastrointestinal problems. Iron replacement and correction of the underlying cause will rapidly relieve the vulvar itch.

Diabetes Mellitus
Late-onset diabetes, especially in an obese patient, may be complicated by an inflammatory intertrigo. This may be limited to the genitocrural region and is usually associated with candidal infection (**18.3**). The lesions usually resolve once the diabetic state has been corrected.

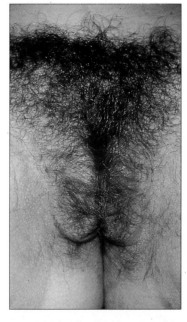

18.1 Lichen simplex, in a patient with chronic pruritus vulvae and iron-deficiency anemia.

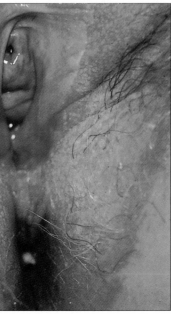

18.2 Eroded, excoriated lichen simplex, in a patient with chronic pruritus vulvae and iron-deficiency anemia.

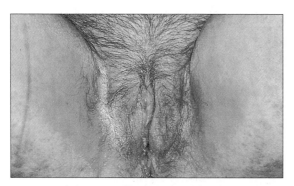

18.3 Intertrigo, complicated by candidiasis in a diabetic.

BEHÇET'S SYNDROME

This condition, first described in 1937 by a Turkish dermatologist, is generally thought to be a viral infection causing genital ulceration. The ulcers are associated with arthritis, ulcerative colitis, thrombophlebitis, skin eruptions, and neurologic problems, and it has been suggested that the condition is an altered immune response to infection in genetically predisposed individuals[3].

Mucocutaneous lesions may be the presenting lesions in Behçet's syndrome, or arise during the course of this multisystem disease. The vulvar lesions are persistent, painful ulcers, which pass deep into the vulvar skin (**18.4**). The labia minora are the most common site for these ulcers. Oral and ocular lesions may also be present. Diagnosis may be difficult in the absence of arthritic, neurologic, or thrombotic disease. The histology of the vulvar ulcers is often non-specific, but may show thrombosed arterioles. Culture and syphilitic tests are negative and a biopsy shows chronic non-specific inflammation.

Systemic steroids or cyclosporin may be indicated if systemic disease is active. Topical steroids provide some relief from the painful vulvar ulcers and may speed up resolution. The lesions usually resolve spontaneously, but result in considerable scarring.

Superpotent topical steroids (clobetasol) may be helpful if applied at the earliest sign of a developing ulcer.

CROHN'S DISEASE

Anogenital manifestations of Crohn's disease are found in up to 30% of patients affected. They may precede intestinal problems by up to several years, and can therefore be a diagnostic problem. Edema is often the first vulvar abnormality (**18.5**), while abscesses, ulcers, sinuses, and fistulae (**18.6**) are the other vulvar complications of Crohn's disease. The lesion may present as a 'knife-cut' ulcer with a thickened edge. It may communicate with the rectum and anus, rendering the patient incontinent due to fistula formation. As Crohn's disease so often mimics other conditions, it is often not diagnosed until biopsies are taken. Non-caseating epithelioid granulomata are found on biopsy, and the differential diagnosis includes other granulomatous disorders, such as sarcoidosis.

Vulvar Crohn's disease usually responds to the medical or surgical management of the intestinal symptoms. When lesions arise unrelated to gut activity, topical or intralesional steroids or topical metronidazole may be beneficial. Occasionally, it is necessary to use wide local excision, including anal resection, to improve the chances of cure. Even so, the risk of recurrence is still high. Anogenital skin lesions are much more rare in ulcerative colitis, but a pustular vegetative eruption in the groins is occasionally present[4].

PYODERMA GANGRENOSUM

'Punched-out' indolent ulcers with a purple edge should arouse suspicion of this disorder. Vulvar lesions are usually multiple and small, and arise on a vasculitic, indurated plaque. However, single lesions

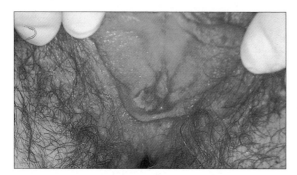

18.4 Behçet's syndrome. Sloughy, shallow, painful vulvar ulcer in Behçet's syndrome.

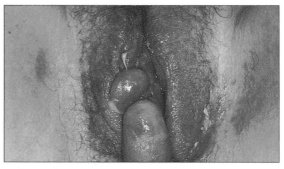

18.5 Crohn's disease. Vulvar edema in Crohn's disease.

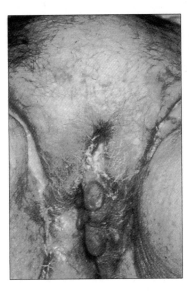

18.6 Crohn's disease. Fissures, fistulae, abscesses and edema in severe vulvar Crohn's disease.

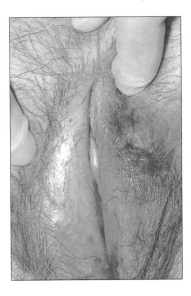

18.7 Pyoderma gangrenosum, in a patient with IgA myeloma.

may be present (**18.7**). As histology shows a non-specific inflammation, a biopsy is unlikely to be helpful.

The ulcers are 'vasculitic' and may be associated with rheumatoid arthritis, inflammatory bowel disease, and myeloma or other lymphoproliferative disorders[5]. Systemic treatment of the underlying disease usually results in resolution of the pyoderma gangrenosum, and the patient should therefore be investigated for diseases known to be associated. Lesions usually respond well to the treatment of an underlying rheumatoid arthritis or ulcerative colitis. However, lesions associated with lymphoproliferative disorders are slower to respond to treatment of the underlying condition, and usually require high doses of systemic steroids. Isolated lesions may respond to intralesional steroid injection.

vulva about 10 days after repeated HSV infections on the face. A detailed history, examination, and biopsy are required to establish the diagnosis. Treatment is for the precipitating cause.

The speed of resolution of drug-induced EM depends on the drug causing the problem, but may be raised by the application of potent topical steroids. Rarely, systemic steroids may be indicated if there is severe mucous membrane involvement in EM, or if EM progresses to toxic epidermal necrolysis[7]. Erythema multiforme following viral infections resolves spontaneously within a week to 10 days. Recurrent attacks of EM after HSV infections may be halted by the immediate use of systemic acyclovir during the HSV prodrome, or continuous administration of suppressive doses.

FIXED DRUG ERUPTION

A patient may react to a drug by always developing a localized skin lesion at the same site after ingestion of the drug. Rarely, this reaction may occur on vulvar skin. Tetracycline and phenolphthalein (found in some laxatives) are both likely to cause fixed drug eruptions (**18.8**). The diagnosis can only be made from a detailed history[6]. The lesion will subside when the drug is withdrawn.

ERYTHEMA MULTIFORME

Erythema multiforme (EM) may result from a drug reaction or may be a complication of HS, mycoplasma, or pregnancy (*see Chapter 8*). Rarely, it is localized to the vulva. In the case shown (**18.9**), the patient developed recurrent blisters and erosions on the

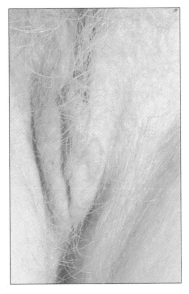

18.8 Fixed drug reaction. Pruritic, blistered patch, occurring on the vulva after each ingestion of tetracycline in a patient with acne rosacea.

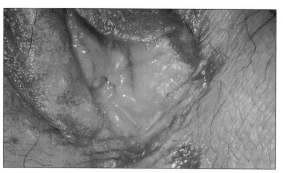

18.9 Erythema multiforme. This recurrent disorder started 10 days after repeated facial herpes simplex.

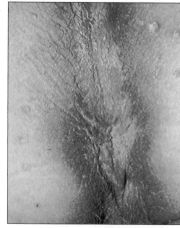

18.10 Ano-genital acanthosis nigricans. This was the presenting feature in a patient with ovarian carcinoma.

ACANTHOSIS NIGRICANS

The vulva and genitocrural region may be involved in any dermatosis which affects flexural sites. In particular, pigmentary disorders tend to affect the vulva. Hyperpigmentation of normal vulvar skin may be part of the flexural pigmentation of Addison's disease or neurofibromatosis. Hyperpigmentation and warty, velvety thickening of the skin should arouse suspicion of acanthosis nigricans (**18.10**). Biopsy is necessary to confirm the diagnosis. Once confirmed, an intensive history, examination, and investigation is indicated, as this disorder is a recognized cutaneous marker of underlying malignancy, especially adenocarcinoma of the stomach[8].

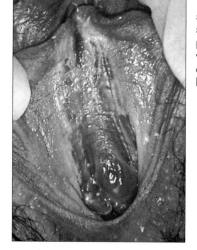

18.11 White sponge nevus syndrome. The patient presented with a white vaginal discharge. She also had oral lesions.

WHITE SPONGE NEVUS SYNDROME

Several inherited mucocutaneous disorders affect the vulva. White sponge nevus is an autosomal-dominant condition with white hyperkeratotic lesions of the oral mucosa and genitalia[9]. Occasionally, the patient may present with symptomless vulvar white patches (**18.11**). Histologically, hyperkeratosis, acanthosis, and vacuolation of the prickle cells confirms the diagnosis. The lesions may clear upon application of a topical antibiotic such as tetracycline mouthwash.

REFERENCES

1. Pincus SH and McKay M. Disorders of the female genitalia. In: Fitzpatrick TB, Eisen AZ, Wolff K, Freedberg IM, Austen KF, (eds.) *Dermatology in general medicine*, 4th ed. New York: McGraw-Hill, 1993, pp 1465–1466.
2. Adams SJ. Iron deficiency and other hematological causes of generalized pruritus. In: Bernhard JD (ed.) *Itch: mechanisms and management of pruritus.* New York: McGraw-Hill, 1994, 243–250.
3. Jorizzo JL. Behçet's disease. In: Fitzpatrick TB, Eisen AZ, Wolff K, Freedberg IM, Austen KF, (eds.) *Dermatology in general medicine,* 4th ed. New York: McGraw-Hill, 1993, pp 2290–2294.
4. Marks JM. The skin and disorders of the alimentary tract. In: Fitzpatrick TB, Eisen AZ, Wolff K, Freedberg IM, Austen KF, (eds.) *Dermatology in general medicine,* 4th ed. New York: McGraw-Hill, 1993, pp 2049–2050.
5. Wolff K and Stingl G. Pyoderma gangrenosum. In: Fitzpatrick TB, Eisen AZ, Wolff K, Freedberg IM, Austen KF, (eds.) *Dermatology in general medicine,* 4th ed. New York: McGraw-Hill, 1993, pp 1171–1182.
6. Blacker KL, Stern RS, Wintroub BU. Cutaneous reactions to drugs. In: Fitzpatrick TB, Eisen AZ, Wolff K, Freedberg IM, Austen KF, (eds.) *Dermatology in general medicine,* 4th ed. New York: McGraw-Hill, 1993, pp 1788.
7. Fritsch PO and Elias PM. Erythema multiforme and toxic epidermal necrolysis. In: Fitzpatrick TB, Eisen AZ, Wolff K, Freedberg IM, Austen KF, (eds.) *Dermatology in general medicine,* 4th ed. New York: McGraw-Hill, 1993, p 585–600.
8. McLean DI and Haynes HA. Cutaneous manifestations of internal malignant disease. In: Fitzpatrick TB, Eisen AZ, Wolff K, Freedberg IM, Austen KF, (eds.) *Dermatology in general medicine,* 4th ed. New York: McGraw-Hill, 1993, pp 2234–2235.
9. Gallagher GT. Biology and pathology of the oral mucosa. In: Fitzpatrick TB, Eisen AZ, Wolff K, Freedberg IM, Austen KF, (eds.) *Dermatology in general medicine,* 4th ed. New York: McGraw-Hill, 1993, pp 1366.

FURTHER READING

Ridley, C. M. (ed.) *The Vulva.* Edinburgh: Churchill Livingstone, 1988: pp.136–211.

19.
Pigmented Lesions of the Vulva

Barbara Rock

INTRODUCTION

About 10–12% of women have pigmented vulvar lesions, as determined by a retrospective analysis of patients seen at a vulvar clinic[1], and a prospective study of a gynecologic practice[2]. Most of these lesions are benign lentigines. Only about 2% of patients have vulvar nevi, and this number decreases with age. Other discrete lesions which can be pigmented include seborrheic keratoses, vascular lesions, genital warts, and malignant tumors such as melanomas, basal cell carcinomas and squamous cell carcinomas. Diffuse hyperpigmentation can also be seen in inflammatory lesions such as lichen simplex chronicus and discoid lupus erythematosus, and in malignant lesions such as squamous cell carcinoma *in situ* and Paget's disease. In short, hyperpigmentation, including normal ethnic variation, is not unusual on the vulva, and differentiating benign from malignant processes is critical for appropriate patient management.

VULVAR NEVI AND MELANOMAS

There has always been particular concern about nevocellular nevi occurring in the vulva, because of the increased risk that a melanoma arising in the vulva seems to carry. Much of this risk is related to the depth, or Breslow level, of the melanoma at the time of diagnosis[3]. Vulvar melanomas tend to be more advanced (i.e. deeper) lesions at the time of diagnosis than melanomas found elsewhere on the body. The depth of the lesion is the single most important prognostic indicator for primary melanoma. Lesions less than 0.85mm deep carry a 10-year survival rate of 95.7%, while lesions deeper than 3.6mm have a 10-year survival rate of 46.0%[4].

It is not yet known if the difference in tumor thickness and prognosis of vulvar lesions are simply related to a delay in diagnosis because of the anatomic site, or if there is a true difference in the biologic behavior of these lesions. Approximately 2–5% of melanomas occur on the vulva, and approximately 8–11% of all vulvar cancers are melanomas[5–7].

Clinically, these lesions are usually deeply pigmented with irregular borders, and share the features of melanomas seen elsewhere on the body. They occur on mucosa as well as on hair-bearing skin of

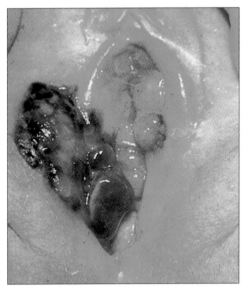

19.1 Melanoma (mucosal). Deeply pigmented and irregular nodules are seen on the labia minora. This is an advanced lesion and therefore the prognosis is grave.

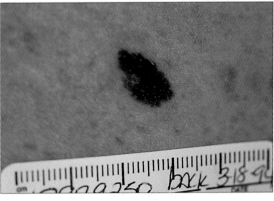

19.2 Melanoma. Typical superficial spreading melanoma with variation in pigmentation and irregular borders. The morphology of these lesions is the same on the skin of the trunk and the vulva.

the vulva. Mucosal melanomas present as flat, very dark, irregularly shaped lesions. Eventually, they develop a nodular component as seen in **19.1**.

Labia majora lesions tend to be of the superficial spreading type (**19.2**), which is the most common form of malignant melanoma. This type of melanoma often has a prolonged radial or horizontal growth phase, during which the lesion expands along the dermoepidermal junction before developing a deep or vertical growth component. The fact that a lesion has been present for a long time is not necessarily reassuring, particularly if there are any signs of enlargement or other change.

Mucosal melanomas may have a distinctive histology, and are referred to as mucosal lentiginous type. Nodular-type melanomas can also occur in both vulvar and mucosal areas and carry the worst prognosis as these lesions tend to develop a deep component quickly.

Benign nevi occurring on the vulva can be junctional (**19.3**), compound (**19.4**), or intradermal. Junctional nevi are typically small, darkly pigmented, slightly raised papules and are found on mucosal and keratinizing skin. They occur from childhood to young adulthood. At times they are indistinguishable from lentigines. Compound nevi contain both a junctional and intradermal component of nevus cells.

They are benign lesions and are generally thought to be a progression from junctional nevi - nevus cells that have 'dropped down' or infiltrated the dermis. Compound nevi are small, dome-shaped, hyperpigmented papules. With time, these lesions tend to lose their junctional component and pigment, and become intradermal. Intradermal nevi are typically small, soft, skin-colored papules that may resemble a skin tag. In general, the morphology and histology of vulvar nevi parallel those of nevi on the torso, as shown in a retrospective histopathologic study comparing 59 vulvar nevi with 50 torso nevi[8].

ATYPICAL MELANOCYTIC NEVUS OF THE VULVA

There appears to be one group of young premenopausal women whose vulvar nevi have distinctive features[8,9]. These lesions (**19.5**) have been called 'atypical melanocytic nevi of the genital (vulvar) type'[10]. They are usually hyperpigmented, papular lesions with indistinct borders, but without the other clinical features of melanoma. Histologically, the lesions are quite unusual, with junctional melanocytic atypia overlying nests of dermal nevus cells. Differentiation from melanoma can be difficult, and evaluation by a dermatopathologist or pathologist with expertise in the diagnosis of melanocytic lesions is required. These lesions are often only distinguished clinically by indistinct borders. The natural history of these lesions has not been determined, though simple excision is usually recommended.

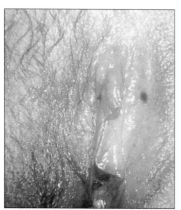

19.3 Junctional nevus. This benign lesion is composed of nevomelanocytes in nests at the dermoepidermal junction and is often associated with lentiginous melanocytic hyperplasia.

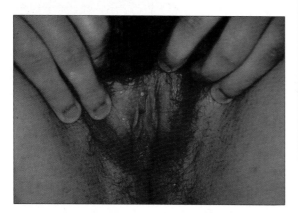

19.4 Compound nevus. Note: ungloved hands in these photographs are the patient's own.

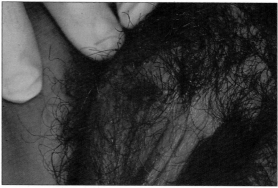

19.5 Atypical melanocytic nevus of the vulva. This lesion was approximately 1cm in size, slightly hyperpigmented, and was flat with a 3mm papule in the central portion. The borders were somewhat indistinct, but the lesion was otherwise unremarkable. This patient had noted the growth of the papular component.

DYSPLASTIC NEVUS

This occurs sporadically and in patients with melanoma or a family history of melanoma (**19.6, 19.7**). The 'atypical mole' is one of several synonyms for dysplastic nevus. These lesions have irregular features compared to normal acquired nevi, including a larger size, a macular and papular component, asymmetry, irregular borders, pigmentation, and a distribution that includes sun-protected skin.

They are generally considered to be a marker for patients who are at increased risk of melanoma. These lesions can occur on the vulva, as well as on other areas of the body. When they occur on the vulva, they share some histologic features with atypical melanocytic nevus of the vulva (*see below*). Excisional biopsy is necessary in most cases to rule out melanoma.

CONGENITAL NEVUS

A congenital nevus (**19.8**) is one that is present at birth, or appears shortly thereafter. These lesions tend to be larger and more irregular in shape than acquired nevi. There is some evidence that the risk of developing malignant melanoma in these lesions is greater than that for acquired nevi, but this is highly controversial. Little research has been done on the biology of congenital vulvar nevi.

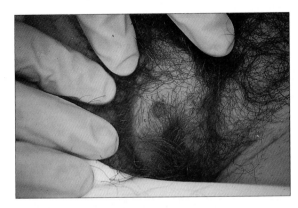

19.6 'Dysplastic' nevus. This lesion on the labia majora was excised and the diagnosis of dysplastic nevus confirmed.

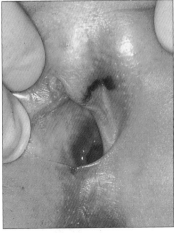

19.8 Congenital nevus.

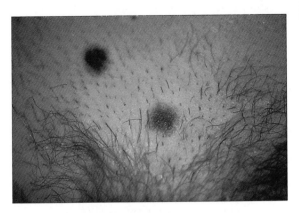

19.7 'Dysplastic' nevus. This patient has multiple dysplastic nevi over her trunk and extremities, as well as a history of malignant melanoma. These lesions resemble melanoma in that they are large and irregularly pigmented. Melanoma was ruled out in this case by excisional biopsy.

LENTIGINES AND VULVAR MELANOSIS

Lentigines are small, less than 5mm wide, hyperpigmented macules, which are found on vulvar skin and mucous membranes in 3.5–7% of patients (**19.9**). Histopathology demonstrates increased pigmentation in the basal cell layer, lentiginous epidermal proliferation, and variable degrees of melanocytic hyperplasia.

The findings of vulvar melanosis (**19.10**) are similar, except that the lesions are larger and may be irregularly shaped, mimicking melanoma[11]. The lesions have similar, if exaggerated, histopathologic features to lentigines, with the additional feature of dermal melanophages. Atypical melanocytes suggestive of melanoma or melanoma precursors are not seen in either lesion. Adequate biopsy is necessary to differentiate vulvar melanosis from melanoma.

HYPERPIGMENTATION ASSOCIATED WITH NON-NEVOMELANOCYTIC LESIONS

Any lesion or cutaneous eruption that has an inflammatory component can result in postinflammatory hyperpigmentation. Lichen simplex chronicus (**19.11**) is the classic example of this, but hyperpigmentation is also a feature of other inflammatory lesions, such as discoid lupus erythematosus (**19.12**). Lichen simplex chronicus is a form of chronic eczema that is often well circumscribed and characterized by lichenification and hyperpigmentation. Discoid lupus erythematosus is a form of cutaneous lupus, in which scarring, follicular plugging, and hypo- or hyperpigmentation are common.

Similarly, some skin-derived, non-melanoma tumors, such as basal cell carcinomas, squamous cell

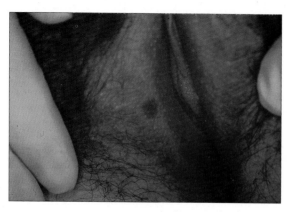

19.9 Lentigo. Typical small, flat, hyperpigmented macule.

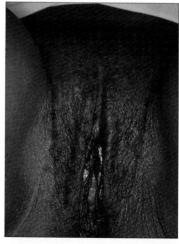

19.11 Lichen simplex chronicus. In this patient, the alteration of skin texture and hyperpigmentation is best seen along the mid-portion of the labia majora.

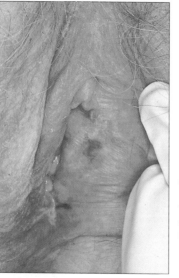

19.10 Vulvar melanosis. This irregularly pigmented lesion on the labia minora shares many clinical features with a dysplastic nevus or melanoma. A second irregularly shaped hyperpigmented lesion is also seen on the mucosa. A biopsy is necessary to confirm the diagnosis of vulvar melanosis.

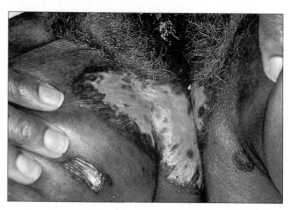

19.12 Discoid lupus. This patient had numerous discoid lesions over the trunk, face and extremities.

carcinomas, VIN, extramammary Paget's disease (**19.13**), and even benign seborrheic keratoses (**19.14**,**19.15**) contain melanocytes and can be pigmented. A seborrheic keratosis is a benign proliferation of keratinocytes and becomes more common with advancing age. Seborrheic keratoses and skin tags are also seen with acanthosis nigricans. The sudden onset of multiple eruptive seborrheic keratoses (sign of Leser-Trélat) may be associated with an internal malignancy, usually an adenocarcinoma.

Hyperpigmentation is a fairly common characteristic of carcinoma *in situ*, and may in fact be the sole clinical clue (**19.16**).

Lastly, some lesions without melanocytes appear to be pigmented, such as vascular lesions and cysts (**19.17**) (*see Chapter 20*).

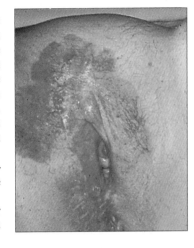

19.13 Extra-mammary Paget's disease. The less common clinical presentation of hyperpigmented, scaly plaques can be seen extending out from the typical, moist, macerated lesions of extramammary Paget's disease.

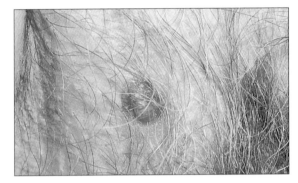

19.14 Seborrheic keratosis. This hyperpigmented, well-circumscribed, 'stuck-on' papule is sometimes confused with melanoma.

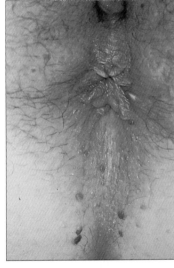

19.15 Multiple seborrheic keratoses. Seborrheic keratoses often occur in large numbers, particularly on the trunk. As in this case, they are benign.

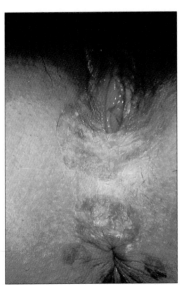

19.16 Carcinoma *in situ*. This patient also had areas of erythema and hyperkeratosis.

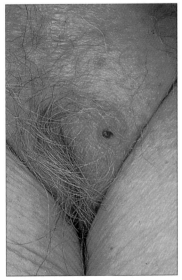

19.17 Epidermoid cyst (epithelial inclusion cyst). These benign cysts filled with necrotic desquamated keratinocytes are not unusual in the vulvar area. They may or may not have a connection to the skin surface. When they do, the cyst contents take on a dark appearance as seen in this lesion.

REFERENCES

1 Friedrich, E. G., Burch, K., and Bahr, J. P. The vulvar clinic: an eight-year appraisal. *Am. J. Obstet. Gynecol.* 1979; **135**: 1036.

2 Rock, B., Hood, A. F., and Rock, J. A. Prospective study of vulvar nevi. *J. Am. Acad. Dermatol.* 1990; **22**: 104.

3 Bradgate, M. G., Rollason, T. P., McConkey, C. C., *et al.* Malignant melanoma of the vulva: a clinicopathologic study of 50 women. *Br. J. Dermatol.* 1990; **97**: 124.

4 Friedman, R. J., Rigel, D. S., Silverman, M. K., *et al.* Malignant melanoma in the 1990s: the continued importance of early detection and the role of the physician examination and self-examination of the skin. *Ca-A Cancer Journal for Clinicians* 1991; **41**(4): 201.

5 Karlen, J. R., Piver, M. S., and Barlow, J. J. Melanoma of the vulva. *Obstet. Gynecol.* 1975; **45**: 181.

6 Morrow, C. P. and DeSaia, P. J. Malignant melanoma of the female genitalia: a clinical analysis. *Obstet. Gynecol. Surv.* 1976; **31**: 233.

7 Ronan, S. G., Eng, A. M., Briele, H. A. *et al.* Malignant melanoma of the female genitalia. *J. Am. Acad. Dermatol.* 1990; **22**: 428.

8 Christtensen, W. N., Friedman, K. J., Woodruff, J. D., *et al.* Histologic characteristics of vulvar nevocellular nevi. *J. Cutan. Pathol.* 1987; **14**: 87.

9 Friedman, R. J. and Ackerman, A. B. Difficulties in the diagnosis of melanocytic nevi on the vulvae of premenopausal women. In: Ackerman, A.B.(ed) *Pathology of Malignant Melanoma.* New York: Masson, 1981: p.119

10 Clark, W. H., Elder, D. E., and Guerry, D. IV. Dysplastic nevi and malignant melanoma. In: Evan, R. Farmer and Antoinette F. Hood (eds) *Pathology of the Skin.* Norwalk, Appleton & Lange, 1990, p.742.

11 Rudolph, R. I. Vulvar melanosis. *J. Am. Acad. Dermatol.* 1990; **23**: 982.

ACKNOWLEDGEMENTS

Figure **19.1** is reproduced from V.R. Tindall *Colour Atlas of Clinical Gynaecology* (Fig 84), Wolfe, London 1981. Figures **19.13** and **19.16** have been reproduced by kind permission of J. Donald Woodruff.

20.
Vulvar Tumors

John M. Monaghan, Ira R. Horowitz, & Marilynne McKay

INTRODUCTION

The superficial vulvar contains skin appendages and a small number of specialized glandular structures, each of which may develop tumors. The vulva has an excellent blood supply and a plethora of nerves. The outer part of the vulva (labia majora) is hair-bearing, with associated apocrine glandular systems. The inner part (labia minora) is covered by stratified squamous epithelium, which blends midway on the inner surface (Hart's Line) into a modification known as mucous membrane (vulvar vestibule) which lacks a granular layer. This non-keratinized surface continues into the vagina. As vulvar tumors may be difficult to differen-tiate from one another, a biopsy is often necessary to establish the diagnosis.

BENIGN TUMORS

There are a variety of benign tumors (**Table 20.1**), of which one group – *the benign pigmented tumors* – has been discussed in *Chapter 19* and so will not be mentioned further.

CONGENITAL TUMORS AND CYSTS

Accessory Breast Tissue
The breast line extends from the anterior border of the axilla, down the chest and abdominal wall, and ends on the vulvar labia majora on each side (**20.1**). Thus, swelling of the vulva, and even breast-milk secretion, may occur during the latter part of preg-

Benign tumors
Pigmented papules and nodules
    See Chapter 19
Congenital tumors and cysts
    Accessory breast tissue
    Hernia
    Mesonephric duct cyst
    Cyst of the canal of Nuck
Cystic tumors
    Vestibular mucous cyst
    Pilonidal cyst or sinus
    Bartholin's cyst or abscess
    Epithelial inclusion cyst
    Lymphangioma
Vascular tumors and swelling
    Hemangioma
    Cherry angioma
    Angiokeratoma
    Pyogenic granuloma
    Endometriosis
    Hematoma
    Edema

Solid papules and tumors
    Skin tag (acrochordon)
    Fibroepithelial polyp
    Neurofibroma
    Syringomata
    Fox-Fordyce disease
    Hidradenoma
'Potentially malignant' tumors
    Fibroma and fibrosarcoma
    Lipoma and liposarcoma
    Granular cell tumor
    Verrucous carcinoma
    Vulvar intraepithelial neoplasia
    (VIN)
Malignant tumors
    Squamous cell carcinoma
    Melanoma
    Basal cell carcinoma
    Adenocarcinoma
    Extramammary Paget's disease
    Adenoid cystic carcinoma
    Sarcoma
    Metastatic tumors

Table 20.1 Vulvar Tumors.

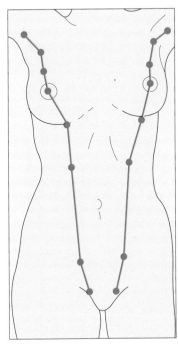

20.1 Breast line.

nancy and into the puerperium. Often, a vestigial nipple is only present as a dark area or small swelling of the skin. However, fully formed nipples with significant amounts of breast tissue have been recorded. It is important to differentiate accessory breast tissue from hidradenoma, labial varicosities, fibroma, or lipoma. The accessory tissue may need to be excised if there are persistent problems. The potential for malignant change clearly exists, though most reports of breast cancer found on the vulva have been secondary from a primary in the breast[1].

Hernia

Inguinal hernias are rare in women. Very rarely, an inguinal hernia may be found to pass down into the upper part of the vulva, where it presents as a small, elongated, unilateral swelling, which is compressible and soft. It is usually not painful, but may become tender due to strangulation or any of the common complications associated with inguinal herniae.

Mesonephric Duct Cysts

During the development of the female fetus, the mesonephric (Wolffian) ducts lie lateral and parallel to the paramesonephric (Müllerian) system (*See Chapter 11*). Remnants of the mesonephric system may remain, resulting in cystic swellings anywhere from the introitus to the broad ligament. Although most commonly found in the upper vagina (Gartner's cysts), it is not unusual to find mesonephric duct cysts on the vulva. They tend to lie laterally, but can be located in various sites, and are commonly confused with the more common vestibular mucous cyst (*see below*). Paramesonephric duct cysts are found only in the vagina; the müllerian system plays no part in the development of the vulva, but this is sometimes a misnomer given to vestibular mucous cysts (*see below*). Treatment is by simple excision if the lesion is symptomatic.

Cyst of the Canal of Nuck

This rare problem may be mistaken for an inclusion cyst or even a hernia. The lesion is small and lies in the inguinal crease or the anterior labia majora, in the line of the round ligament remnant as it enters the upper part of the vulva on the lateral side. The diagnosis is usually made following excision of the cyst.

CYSTIC TUMORS

Vestibular Mucous Cysts

These are usually confined to the vestibular ring of the introitus and are probably more common than is thought. They are not infrequently seen in the newborn, but are less commonly diagnosed in the adult. These dysontogenetic cysts are usually asymptom-

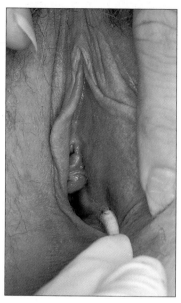

20.2 Vestibular mucous cyst. This asymptomatic lesion was found on incidental examination of a patient with recurrent candidiasis. Note: ungloved fingers are the patient's own.

atic and ignored by both patient and physician. The cysts lie between the hymenal ring and the outer part of the labia minora (**20.2**), and are thought to be caused by obstruction of the ducts of the small vestibular glands. They may be yellow, bluish, or skincolored, and usually have a translucent appearance. Similar mucous cysts may also arise in close relationship to the urethra, where they may occasionally cause obstruction or diversion of urinary flow. Treatment is by simple excision if the cyst is symptomatic or the patient wants it removed.

Pilonidal Cysts or Sinuses

These lesions begin as abscesses that develop from a foreign-body inflammatory reaction to hair within the dermis. The hair may be from a ruptured dermoid cyst or an ingrown follicle. The most common location is in the lower sacrococcygeal area, but they may occur on the vulva, usually around the clitoris but sometimes on the mons pubis or perineum. Clinically, these are red papules that frequently erode and drain, forming a chronic sinus tract. The entire sinus tract must be excised to prevent recurrence.

Bartholin's Cyst or Abscess

Bartholin's glands are bilateral and lie posterolaterally in the introitus at 5:00 and 7:00. The ducts secrete into the posterior vestibule at the base of the hymen, and provide a degree of lubrication – though most sexual lubrication in sexually experienced women is from vaginal secretions. Occasionally, the ostium of a Bartholin's gland may become obstructed, causing the gland and duct to swell to a large size. The entire gland can be grasped between finger and thumb (**20.3**) when this occurs. If the gland is not infected, the swelling is painless.

While the fluid contained within the Bartholin's cyst may be spontaneously released, it is often necessary to release the contents surgically. A standard procedure is that of marsupialization, whereby the cyst is deroofed (**20.4**) and the edges are carefully oversewn so as to generate a functioning duct (**20.5**)[2]. An alternative method is to make a small incision in the roof of the cyst and insert a Word catheter (or trimmed-off short pediatric Foley catheter), which is then inflated and allowed to remain in place for several weeks[3,4] (**20.6**). Complete excision of the cyst is occasionally performed when there is recurrent painful obstruction. In cases where infection has been the cause of the obstruction, a combination of antibiotics and surgical drainage gives the best results.

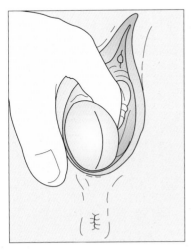

20.3 Marsupialization of Bartholin's cyst. A right-sided Bartholin's cyst is shown being elevated by introducing the index finger into the lower vagina. The line of incision is shown.

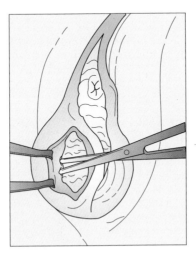

20.4 Marsupialization of Bartholin's cyst. The Bartholin's cyst is being released from the overlying skin and excess skin removed.

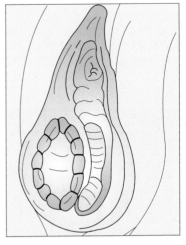

20.5 Marsupialization of Bartholin's cyst. The edges of the marsupialized cyst have been oversewn so that the secreting part of the gland can be preserved. Once healing is complete the defect will remain as a small hole through which secretions can pass.

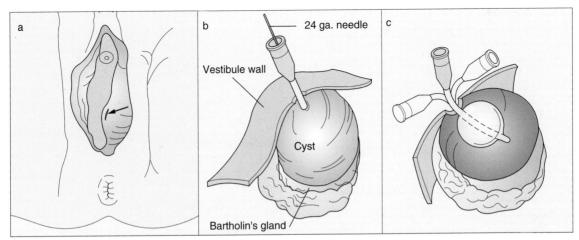

20.6 Inflatable catheter for Bartholin's cyst. This shows the inflatable bulb-tipped catheter used to treat Bartholin's cysts and abscesses. (a) An arrow indicates the location for a stab wound in a cyst or abscess. (b) Insertion of the catheter in the stab wound. (c) Inserted catheter inflated with 2–4ml of water.

Epithelial Inclusion Cysts

Also called sebaceous, keratinous, or epidermoid cysts, these lesions are very common on the labia majora and sometimes minora (**20.7**). From time to time, they may become very extensive, making diagnosis more difficult (**20.8**). The cysts are lined by keratinizing squamous epithelium and are filled with a cheesy white accumulation of waxy secretions and cell debris. In contrast to lesions on the scalp, vulvar cysts tend to be small, multiple, and grouped. They may be recognized by a yellowish appearance and knobbly feel. If the patient is symptomatic or bothered by the appearance, simple excision is appropriate. Cysts will recur after incision and drainage unless the cyst wall is removed.

Lymphangiomata

These localized dilations and ectasias of lymphatic vessels may appear at any age, though one form (lymphangioma circumscriptum) typically develops in childhood. They usually appear as papules or nodules, from which a clear or milky fluid may drain. Diagnosis is made on biopsy and observation of the white lymphatic fluid (**20.9, 20.10**)

VASCULAR TUMORS AND SWELLING

Hemangiomas

Three forms of hemangiomas may be found on the vulva. The *cherry angioma* is extremely common, and

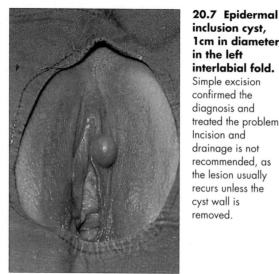

20.7 Epidermal inclusion cyst, 1cm in diameter, in the left interlabial fold. Simple excision confirmed the diagnosis and treated the problem. Incision and drainage is not recommended, as the lesion usually recurs unless the cyst wall is removed.

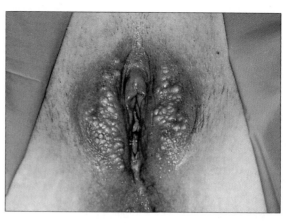

20.8 Multiple sebaceous cysts on both labia majora. The patient wished removal of the cysts, and a simple excision of both affected areas provided a satisfactory cosmetic result.

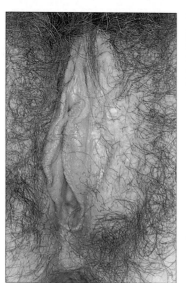

20.9 Lymphangiomata on the left labium majus. Note the white nodular lesions.

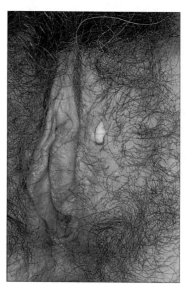

20.10 Biopsy of lymphangiomata. The lymphangiomata shown in **20.9** were easily compressible and drained typical white lymphatic fluid on biopsy.

is a small dark-red papule usually 2–3mm in diameter (**20.11**). Cherry angiomas are discrete lesions which are usually scattered over the trunk; they tend to increase in number with age and are most numerous in the fifth and sixth decades. Treatment is unnecessary.

Angiokeratomas are also fairly common, and since they occur mostly on the vulva they are more likely to be encountered in a women's clinic. Lesions are usually multiple, dark red to almost black, and the diagnosis is confirmed when they blanch with pressure (**20.12**). They may be more prominent in pregnancy and with venous stasis. The histologic architecture shows interlacing layers of squamous cells with blood-filled spaces.

Pyogenic granulomas are capillary tumors which usually arise as the result of trauma. Oral gingival les- ions are thought to be most common during pregnancy, but these tumors may arise at any time and at any location on the body (*see also* **3.15**, **3.16**). Excisional biopsy is recommended, as these lesions may mimic an amelanotic melanoma.

Endometriosis

Very rarely, ectopic endometrium may be found on the vulva – it is more often seen on the cervix or in the vagina. The commonest etiology is for the endometrium to be implanted at the time of surgery on the perineum. It typically presents as a small mass which is cyclically uncomfortable. The surface appearance is often blue or darkly colored, but deep lesions may be flesh-colored (**20.13**, **20.14**). Incision may occasionally produce old blood. Diagnosis and treatment are usually by local excision.

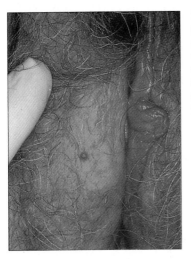

20.11 Cherry angioma, a common benign vascular tumor which can appear anywhere on the trunk.

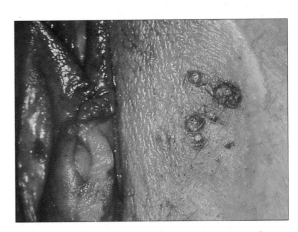

20.12 Angiokeratomas, commonly seen on the vulva or scrotum.

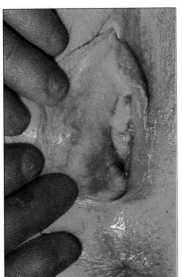

20.13 Endometriosis of the labium majus. There is a small nodule with a dimple on the right side.

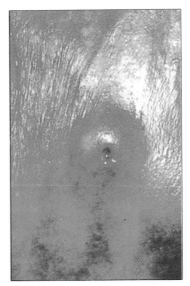

20.14 Close-up of nodule shown in 20.13, showing cyclic drainage site for blood-tinged fluid when ovulation was not being suppressed.

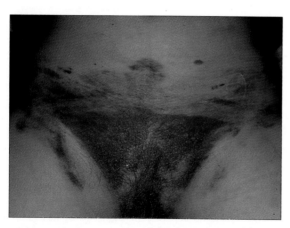

20.15 Ecchymoses and vulvar hematoma after abdominal liposuction (note bilateral sutures on incisions on lower abdomen). Extravasation of blood to dependent areas may cause marked discoloration even when vulvar trauma has not occurred.

Medications
Bacitracin
Benzocaine
Gentamicin
Neomycin
Penicillin
Lindane
Additives, preservatives, fragrances
Acetic acid
Many alcohols
Balsam of Peru
Benzoic acid
Cinnamic aldehyde, acid
Formaldehyde
Lanolin
Menthol
Parabens
Polyethylene glycol
Polysorbate 60
Sodium benzoate
Other
Animal dander
Hair
Latex
Nickel
Placenta
Saliva
Semen

*From von Krogh, G. and Maibach, H.I. The contact urticaria syndrome – 1982. *Semin. Dermatol.* 1982; **1**: 59.

Table 20.2 Causes of Contact Urticaria.

Hematoma

Usually the result of trauma or intraoperative bleeding, ecchymoses of the vulva can cause extensive purple-black discoloration of the vulva (**20.15**). Vulvar hematomas can also develop postoperatively if complete hemostasis has not been achieved; extravasation through the soft tissue occurs rapidly, often reaching onto the thigh. Hematomas of the vulva can also develop after relatively minor trauma. Accidents such as straddle injuries or split-legged falls will cause disruption of vulvar small vessels, particularly of the erectile tissue deep in the labia majora. The extravasated blood rapidly expands the loose areolar tissue of the labia, causing considerable swelling. The swelling ceases when the tension within it reaches that of the arterial blood supply; this tense swelling is exquisitely painful and often requires powerful analgesia.

Conservative treatment consists in the application of ice-packs as soon as possible. If this is not effective, surgical evacuation of the hematoma may then be necessary. Since it is often difficult to identify single bleeding points, insertion of a vacuum drain may be required. If swelling is extensive, urinary flow may be compromised; a urinary catheter provides relief and keeps the area clean.

Edema

An edematous vulva can reach remarkable proportions. The condition is most commonly found as a complication of generalized abdominal edema, such as that associated with cardiac or liver failure. Obstruction of vulvar lymphatic drainage, due to surgical extirpation of the groin lymph glands or their massive involvement by tumor, will cause an irreversible enlargement of the entire vulva, often obstructing the entrance to the vagina.

Acute local edema or angioedema may be due to an immunologically mediated contact urticaria - the most important substance to consider is latex in examining gloves, condoms, and diaphragms (**Table 20.2**); anaphylaxis has been reported with severe sensitivity. Inflammation due to *Candida* infection can also produce an edematous appearance (**20.16**). The application of topical agents typically produces the complaint of burning on inflamed skin, but this is not an allergic reaction.

Chronic edema can cause the vulva to acquire a verrucous appearance which is sometimes mistaken for genital warts (**20.17**); lymphatic leakage may be mistaken for herpetic blisters. Crohn's disease of the bowel, hidradenitis suppurativa, and infestation of the lymphatics by filariasis may also present with vulvar edema.

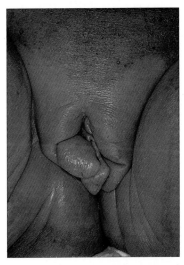

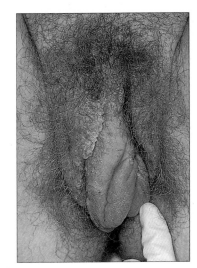

20.17 Chronic lymphedema after bilateral lymphadenectomy for cancer. This young woman suffered significant discomfort sitting down, and distortion of the vulva made coitus difficult (gloved finger is at inlet). The papillary appearance of the anterior right labium majus is typical of chronic lymphedema (although the patient had been told this was genital warts). The area was easily traumatized; lymphatic drainage from abrasion sites had also been misdiagnosed as herpes simplex.

20.16 Vulvar edema in nursing home patient with chronic intertrigo. Poor circulation contributes to chronic vulvar edema.

SOLID TUMORS

Skin Tags and Fibroepithelial Polyps

Skin tags (acrochordons) are a common finding on almost any skin surface (**20.18**). They are small soft filiform papules, ranging from 1 to 2mm diameter and 3 - 5mm in length in the anogenital region; they are smaller and more numerous in the axillae and around the neck. Pigmentation is variable, depending on the skin color of the patient. They have no medical significance, and are usually only removed for diagnosis or if they grow to any significant size. Management is essentially cosmetic, and excision using scissors is effective.

Fibroepithelial polyps (soft fibromas) are more common in the anogenital region. The fibrofatty and muscular layers of the vulva and ischiorectal fossae can give rise to quite enormous fleshy soft tumors (**20.19**). Clinically, these are similar to neurofibromas; histology makes the diagnosis. The stalk of a large polypoid lesion may become twisted, causing spontaneous necrosis with swelling.

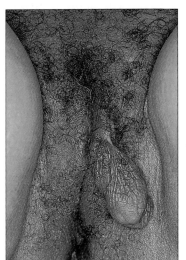

20.18 Skin tag. This skin tag demonstrates the typical pedunculated nature of this benign tumor.

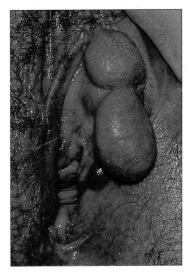

20.19 A bilobed fibrous lipoma of the left labium majus. Slow growth over many years suggested its benign nature, which was confirmed on excision. A small inclusion cyst is also present below the lipoma.

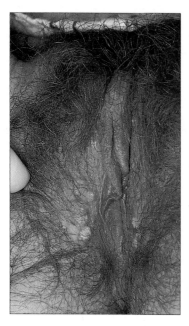

20.20 Multiple syringomata on both labia majora. The patient complained of itching and irritation from the larger lesions on the right, which were successfully excised under local anesthesia.

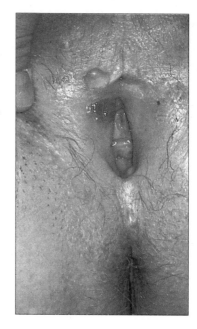

20.21 A small hidradenoma is seen at the right side of the vulva which also shows marked atrophic change in a postmenopausal patient.

Neurofibroma

Solitary neurofibromas resemble fibroepithelial polyps (*see above*) and can be found anywhere on the body. Neurofibromatosis (Von Recklinghausen's) produces the classic findings of café au lait spots, dermal neurofibromas, and subcutaneous nodules. Perineal and axillary freckling are virtually pathognomic for neurofibromatosis and can be seen in childhood. Excision is only required when nodules interfere with urinary function or coitus due to their position or size.

Syringomata

These benign tumors of the eccrine sweat glands usually appear as clusters, especially on the face and lower eyelids. Vulvar lesions are smooth flesh-colored papules 2–5mm in diameter. They occur on the hairy part of the vulva (**20.20**), and since they are usually asymptomatic, the diagnosis may be missed, accounting for the rarity of reports in the literature.

Fox-Fordyce Disease

These pruritic papules are related to the apocrine glands of hair follicles, and occur primarily on the mons pubis, labia majora, and axillae. The condition is more likely to occur in black-skinned individuals, and it develops after puberty. Fox-Fordyce papules resemble syringomata, but they are smaller, darker, and more pruritic. High-potency topical steroids may be helpful in treating secondary lichen simplex chronicus. The condition regresses with menopause.

Hidradenoma

Hidradenoma papilliferum is a rare tumor of Caucasian women, arising from the apocrine portion of the sweat glands. Although in the past it had been branded as malignant, it is in fact a benign tumor. The usual presentation is that of a small, 1cm-diameter mass arising from the labia or the interlabial sulcus (**20.21**). The lesion surface is usually intact, but if ulcerated it can generate significant bleeding. Treatment is usually excision for diagnosis.

'POTENTIALLY MALIGNANT' TUMORS

The tumors listed below are most often benign, and it is difficult to distinguish malignant lesions without histologic confirmation. The examiner is advised to proceed with caution when tumors are reported to be changing appearance or increasing in size.

FIBROMA AND FIBROSARCOMA

Two different types of these tumors may be seen on the vulva. The first type resembles a fibroepithelial polyp, but is firm rather than soft on palpation, while the second type is a sessile, firm nodule. Both are asymptomatic, flesh-colored, and slow growing. Malignant lesions are not clinically different and may develop at any age. Excision is curative for benign lesions, but malignant lesions often recur.

LIPOMA AND LIPOSARCOMA

These fatty tumors are hamartomas of the subcutaneous tissue. They are typically asymptomatic and slow growing; treatment is seldom necessary. Fast-growing lesions should be biopsied to rule out liposarcoma. The latter soft-tissue malignancy arises from intermuscular fascial planes rather than from a lipoma. Liposarcomas are more firm on palpation than lipomas.

GRANULAR CELL TUMORS

These rare neoplasms are more common in African-American women. They are usually solitary and occur in early adult life. Most genital lesions that have been reported are on the vulva, usually the labia majora. They are round, firm lesions averaging 2–4cm in diameter; they may be either smooth or hyperkeratotic. Histologic examination shows large cells containing granule-filled, pale cytoplasm; the granules are periodic acid-Schiff (PAS) positive. Lesions with histologic atypia may metastasize, as can some lesions which are histologically benign[5].

VERRUCOUS CARCINOMA

Although this tumor can grow to a remarkable size, it is commonly regarded as an essentially benign growth (**20.22**). In the past, the condition has been called the 'giant condyloma of Buschke-Löwenstein' and it has been included here because of its propensity to spread by local 'pushing' margins and occasional reports of metastasis to regional lymph nodes. Some gynecologic oncologists believe that condylomas and verrucous carcinomas are separate lesions[6], though recent studies have found a close association with human papillomavirus type 6. In the spectrum of squamous cancer of the vulva, verrucous carcinoma lies toward the benign end. Although it has often been stated that verrucous carcinomas can become anaplastic if treated by irradiation, there have been few case reports.

Treatment

Wide local excision is required to treat these lesions. Margins should be evaluated to ensure complete excision. Lymphadenectomy is indicated for palpable and suspicious lymph nodes. Radiotherapy, as noted above, is unnecessary and inappropriate[7].

VULVAR INTRAEPITHELIAL NEOPLASIA

Vulvar intraepithelial neoplasia (VIN) is categorized as mild (1), moderate (2), severe or carcinoma *in situ* (3)[8]. The VIN classification was introduced by the International Society for the Study of Vulvovaginal Disease to replace the many other names widely in use. Bowen's disease, erythroplasia of Queyrat, and carcinoma *in situ* simplex are all included in VIN 3. Bowenoid papulosis, another form of VIN, is often characterized by its pigmented lesions (**20.23**). Both white and red lesions occur and represent other vari-

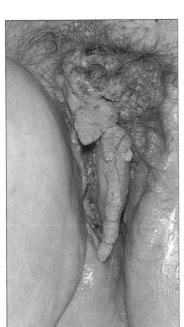

20.22 Verrucous carcinoma. A relatively small example of verrucous carcinoma showing the smooth pushing edge of the lesion. Excision biopsy was adequate therapy in this case.

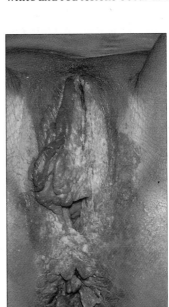

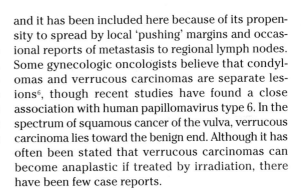

20.23 Widespread vulvar intraepithelial neoplasia (VIN) was found to hide multiple areas of early invasive cancer of the vulva. The patient also had cervical intraepithelial neoplasia (CIN) 3, and 10 years later she developed a primary invasive vaginal cancer. Multifocal disease of this type is not uncommon and may represent a 'field effect' of human papillomavirus (HPV) infection.

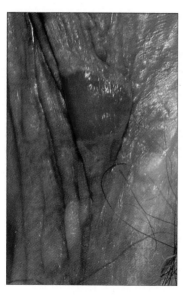

20.24 Vulvar intraepithelial neoplasia (VIN). A typical example of VIN of the 'red type'. The diagnosis can only be made on biopsy. Biopsy of the raised white area also confirmed VIN.

neoplasia of the cervix, vagina, and perianal regions. Human papillomavirus infections have been associated with VIN[8,9]. It is controversial whether or not VIN is a precursor of vulvar carcinoma.

Treatment

If no evidence of an invasive lesion is present, VIN may be treated with the following modalities: simple vulvectomy, skinning vulvectomy, local excision, topical 5-fluorouracil, cryosurgery, carbon dioxide (CO_2) laser ablation, and ultrasonic surgical aspiration. The most commonly used and accepted techniques are wide local excision and CO_2 laser ablation.

MALIGNANT TUMORS

Invasive squamous cell cancer of the vulva represents between 5 and 8% of all female genital cancers; it is much less common than cervical cancer and occurs in older patients. In recent years, the proportion has been increasing due to a continuing decline in invasive cancer of the cervix and a steadily increasing proportion of elderly women in the population.

Symptomatology

Most patients present complaining of itching, irritation, or soreness on the vulva, often of many years' duration. A lump (**20.25**) or slight bleeding may have been noticed, but these are less commonly reported than irritation or itching. The disease is commonly characterized by delay; both by the patient who self medicates or ignores lesions, or by the healthcare provider who prescribes repeatedly without examining the patient. Embarrassment by one or both is often contributory. As a consequence, all too often the cancer is well advanced by the time the patient presents (**20.26**).

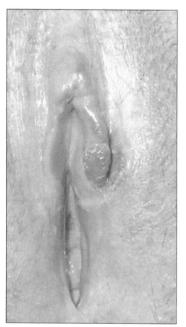

20.25 A small nodule of carcinoma at the lower part of the labia minora. Epithelial whitening, obliteration of the clitoral hood, and loss of vulvar architecture are consistent with the diagnosis of lichen sclerosus. Despite the size of this tumor, the lymph nodes in the groins contained carcinoma - the size of a tumor does not always reflect the extent of tumor spread.

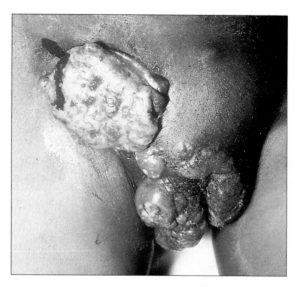

20.26 A massive metastasizing vulvar carcinoma in a young black woman. Palliative surgery was performed to improve the quality of life.

SQUAMOUS CARCINOMA

About 90–95% of cancers of the vulva are squamous. The mean age for presentation is in the late seventh decade, though the age range is wide, and patients may have vulvar cancers as early as the third decade (i.e. in their early 20s). Most squamous cancers presenting in older women are unifocal (**20.25**) and are often preceded by years of vulvar irritation or lichen sclerosus (*see Chapter 16*), though the latter condition is not considered a precursor.

Treatment

Cancer of the vulva should be managed in a specialist center where a gynecologic oncologist can deliver the best quality care for the patient. In the past decade, there has been a trend toward conservative management of patients with vulvar carcinoma, with special consideration of cosmetic appearance and sexual function, especially in the younger patient.

Stage I (FIGO) carcinoma, with lesions less than 2cm in diameter and less than or equal to 1mm stromal invasion, should be treated with a local wide radical excision. Lateral lesions with more than 1mm stromal invasion should be treated with radical hemivulvectomy and ipsilateral inguinal femoral lymphadenectomy[10]. Midline lesions should be treated with radical vulvectomy and bilateral inguinal femoral lymphadenectomy. In Stage I lesions, the bilateral lymphadenectomy can be performed through separate incisions rather than the *en bloc* resection described below.

For Stages II and III (FIGO), the *en bloc*, 'butterfly', or three-incision approach are effective methods of therapy. It is rare to perform a pelvic-node dissection as part of primary therapy for vulvar carcinoma. Postoperative pelvic radiation has been proven effective in treating patients with positive femoral lymph nodes[11,12].

Radiotherapy to the groin and pelvic side wall is recommended where two or more nodes are involved, or where there is complete replacement of the node or capsular rupture. Cure rates for vulvar cancer in the major centers are now extremely good, with node-negative and node-positive patients achieving 94 and 62% five-year survival respectively.

FIGO Stage IV patients have traditionally undergone radical vulvectomy, pelvic exenteration, and bilateral inguinal femoral lymphadenectomy. Patients with advanced stages are now offered neoadjuvant radiation or chemoradiation prior to surgical excision. This procedure has enabled oncologists to use less radical surgery[13].

MELANOMA

This rare condition is the second most common vulvar malignancy; it occurs predominantly in postmenopausal Caucasian women[14]. Unlike the previous vulvar malignancies, melanoma is staged by the depth of the lesion[15] (*see Chapter 19*). Melanomas occur most often on the labia majora, clitoris, and labia minora. They can arise *de novo* or from a pre-existing junctional nevus on the skin or mucous membrane. About 50% of vulvar melanomas are of the superficial spreading variety (**20.27**). Nodular melanoma is a protuberant tumor which often exhibits both melanotic and amelanotic elements (**20.28**). Amelanotic lesions are relatively more common on the vulva, and may present with ulceration, crusting, and bleeding.

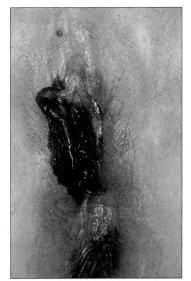

20.27 Vulvar melanoma. A very clear area of dense pigmented tissue with an irregular edge was in fact diagnosed as an '*in situ*' melanoma. Wide local excision produced a cure of the tumor.

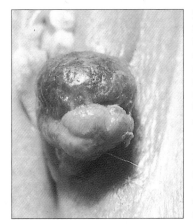

20.28 Vulvar melanoma. This unusual example of a combined melanotic and amelanotic melanoma was found to have extensive involvement of the inguinal nodes. The metastases represented both melanotic and amelanotic elements.

Treatment

Lesions of less than 0.75mm invasion should be treated with wide local radical excision with 2cm margins. Lymph node excision is not required, as the five-year survival rate is 98%. The outcome is directly related to the histologic depth of the lesion at the time of excision. A depth of invasion of less than 1.5mm has a good prognosis with wide local resection. Small lateralizing lesions of more than 0.75mm invasion must be treated with a radical hemivulvectomy, with ipsilateral inguinal femoral lymph adenectomy. Radical surgery for large lesions (*en bloc* radical vulvectomy and bilateral inguinal femoral lymphadenectomy[16]), though rarely curative, may increase survival time, and radiation may provide helpful palliative treatment.

BASAL CELL CARCINOMA

Accounting for less than 5% of vulvar cancers, basal cell carcinoma of the vulva has the same characteristics as tumors occurring in other parts of the body. Vulvar basal cell carcinoma is more prevalent in Caucasian women over the age of 50, and lesions usually occur on hair-bearing skin. The presenting lesion is usually a dome-shaped nodule or plaque with a small rolled edge ('rodent ulcer'). There is surprisingly little pain and discomfort, but itching may be a complaint. Basal cell carcinomas are further discussed in appendix A (page 164).

Treatment

Basal cell carcinoma is easily managed by wide local excision. An excision biopsy with good margins may not only be diagnostic, but curative as well. For elderly patients with large lesions, radiation therapy can be an effective modality.

ADENOCARCINOMA (BARTHOLIN'S GLAND)

This rare cancer is generally found in association with Bartholin's gland. It is characterized by the appearance of a relatively large mass lying deep to the vulvar and vaginal skin, often with only a small area of ulceration. The diagnosis is commonly made during the surgical treatment of a Bartholin's cyst. Solid, suspicious material is found, which histology proves to be an adenocarcinoma. Lymph node metastasis is found in 37% of Bartholin carcinomas[17,18]. The condition is treated in the same way as a squamous tumor, with great care being taken to achieve an adequate margin in resection of the vulva.

EXTRAMAMMARY PAGET'S DISEASE

This malignancy results from neoplastic secretory, glandular adenocarcinoma cells arising in the vulvar epidermis. Vulvar Paget's may have migrated from a local tumor or be a metastasis from a distant neoplasm such as the breast. It is rare (less than 0.2% of all vulvar carcinomas), but because of its similarity to benign vulvar dermatoses, it should be a diagnostic consideration when lesions fail to clear with appropriate therapy. The patient presents with a slowly growing eroded velvety plaque (**20.29**) which may be sore, but is rarely as itchy as typical dermatitic lesions. Histology confirms the diagnosis and a search for adjacent or distant neoplasm should be made[19].

Treatment

The preferred treatment is wide local excision with 3cm margins and depth of resection to Colles' fascia. Recurrent *in situ* disease may be treated conservatively with topical bleomycin or 5-fluorouracil, CO_2 laser vaporization, or systemic retinoids[20].

If there is stromal invasion of underlying sweat glands, the surgeon should perform a radical hemivulvectomy and ipsilateral inguinal femoral lymph node dissection.

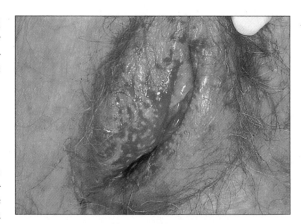

20.29 Vulvar (extramammary) Paget's disease.
The similarity to vulvar eczema may delay diagnosis for months or years. No local or distant neoplasm was found in this patient.

ADENOID CYSTIC CARCINOMA

This rare variant is characterized by a tendency to spread much more widely than at first appears by a process of subdermal infiltration (**20.30**). The normal margin for acceptable clearance of 1–2cm may have to be significantly extended if the local disease is to be controlled effectively. The extent of this lesion is often underestimated. It is essential that a very wide excision is performed because there is a high risk of recurrent disease if this is not done. Survival is decreased compared to squamous cell carcinoma (five-year survival is 5.5% compared to 62.3%, respectively[21]). Extensive surgery should consist in a radical vulvectomy and inguinal femoral lymph node dissection.

SARCOMA

Sarcomas of the vulva are extraordinarily rare, representing 1–2% of vulvar cancers. A wide variety of sarcomas have been described, including leiomyosarcomas, angiosarcomas, fibrosarcomas, neurofibrosarcomas, liposarcomas, and rhabdomyosarcomas. Wide local excision is the mainstay of therapy.

SECONDARY MALIGNANT TUMORS OF THE VULVA

Cancers may spread to the vulva from the anus, vagina, cervix, endometrium, ovary (**20.31**), breast, kidney, and thyroid.

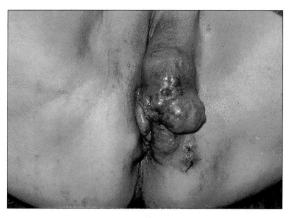

20.30 Adenoid cystic carcinoma. In contrast to the superficial lesions of Paget's disease, this adenoid cystic cancer undermines the epithelium to a far greater extent than is apparent. This lesion had invaded the pubic ramus as well as the bladder and required exenterative surgery to treat.

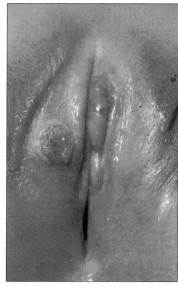

20.31 Secondary ovarian tumor. This small tumor occurred in a patient who had been treated one year previously for ovarian cancer. Although it clinically resembled a primary vulvar lesion, histology revealed it to be identical with the previously resected ovarian primary.

References

1 Garcia, J. J., Verkauf, B. S., Hochberg, C. J., *et al.* Aberrant breast tissue of the vulva. *Obstet. Gynecol.* 1978; **52**: 225–228.

2 Friedrich, E. G. Jr. *Surgical Procedures in Vulvar Disease.* 2nd ed. Philadelphia: W. B. Saunders, 1983: p.68.

3 Word, B. Office treatment of cyst and abscess of Bartholin's gland duct. *South Med. J.* 1968; **61**: 514–518.

4 Friedrich, E. G. Jr. *Surgical Procedures in Vulvar Disease.* 2nd ed. Philadelphia: W. B. Saunders, 1983: p.70.

5 Majmudar, B., Castellano, P. Z., Wilson, R. W., *et al.* Granular cell tumors of the vulva. *J. Reprod. Med.* 1990; **35**: 90.

6 Partridge, E. E., Murad, T., Shingleton, H. M., *et al.* Verrucous lesions of the female genitalia. II. Verrucous carcinoma. *Am. J. Obstet. Gynecol.* 1980; **137**: 419–424.

7 Kaufman, R. H. and Woodruff, J. D. The vulvar dystrophies, atypias, carcinomata *in situ*: an invitational symposium. Historical background in developmental stages of the new nomenclature. *J. Reprod. Med.* 1976; **17**: 132–136.

8 Crum, C. P., Braun, L. A., Shah, K. V., *et al.* Vulvar intraepithelial neoplasia: correlation of nuclear DNA content and the presence of a human papilloma virus (HPV) structural antigen. *Cancer* 1982; **49**: 468–471.

9 Gross, G., Hagedorn, M., Ikenberg, H., *et al.* Bowenoid papulosis: presence of human papillomavirus (HPV) structural antigens and of HPV 16-related DNA sequences. *Arch. Dermatol.* 1985; **121**: 858–863.

10 Stehman, F. B., Bundy, B. N., Dvoretsky, P. M., *et al.* Early stage I carcinoma of the vulva treated with ipsilateral superficial inguinal lymphadenectomy and modified radical hemivulvectomy: a prospective study of the Gynecologic Oncology Group. *Obstet. Gynecol.* 1992; **79**: 490–497.

11 Burrell, M. O., Franklin, E. W. III, Campion, M. J., *et al.* The modified radical vulvectomy with groin dissection: an eight-year experience. *Am. J. Obstet. Gynecol.* 1988; **159**: 715–722.

12 Cavanagh, D., Roberts, W. S., Bryson, S. C., *et al.* Changing trends in the surgical treatment of invasive carcinoma of the vulva. *Surg. Gynecol. Obstet.* 1986; **162**: 164–168.

13 Berek, J. S., Heaps, J. M., Fu, Y. S., *et al.* Concurrent cisplatin and 5-fluorouracil chemotherapy and radiation therapy for advanced-stage squamous carcinoma of the vulva. *Gynecol. Oncol.* 1991; **42**: 197–201.

14 Ronan, S. G., Eng, A. M., Briele, H. A., *et al.* Malignant melanoma of the female genitalia. *J. Am. Acad. Dermatol.* 1990; **22**: 428.

15 Look, K. Y., Roth, L. M., and Sutton, G. P. Vulvar melanoma reconsidered. *Cancer* 1993; **72**: 143.

16 Podratz, K. C., Gaffey, T. A., Symmonds, R. E., *et al.* Melanoma of the vulva: an update. *Gynecol. Oncol.* 1983; **16**: 153–168.

17 Leuchter, R. S., Hacker, N. F., Voet, R. L., *et al.* Primary carcinoma of the Bartholin gland: a report of 14 cases and review of the literature. *Obstet. Gynecol.* 1982; **60**: 361.

18 Copeland, L. J., Sneigen, W., Gershenson, D. M., *et al.* Bartholin gland carcinoma. *Obstet. Gynecol.* 1986; **67**: 794–801.

19 Sitaklin, C. and Ackerman, A. B. Mammary and extramammary Paget's disease (groin, vulva, perianal). *Am. J. Dermatopathol.* 1985; **7**: 335–340.

20 Stacy, D., Burrell, M. O., and Franklin, E. W. III. Extramammary Paget's disease of the vulva and anus: use of intraoperative frozen–section margins. *Am. J. Obstet. Gynecol.* 1986; **155**: 519–523.

21 Underwood, J. W., Adcock, L. L., and Okagaki, T. Adenosquamous carcinoma of skin appendages (adenoid squamous cell carcinoma, pseudoglandular squamous cell carcinoma, adenocanthoma of sweat gland of Lever) of the vulva. A clinical and ultrastructural study. *Cancer* 1978; **42**: 1851–1858.

ACKNOWLEDGEMENTS

Figures **20.13**, **20.14** and **20.25** are reproduced from V.R. Tindall Colour Atlas of Clinical Gynaecology (Figs 57, 58 and 90), Wolfe, London 1981. Figure 20.6 has been reproduced with permission from: Word, B. New instrument for office treatment of cysts and abscesses of Bartholin's gland. *J.A.M.A.* 1964; 190: 777.

Appendix A
Differential Diagnosis of the Vulvar Ulcer

Marilynne McKay

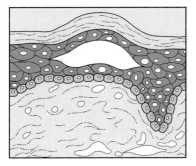

1 Blister (when the roof is lost, an erosion remains).

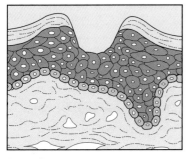

2 Erosion (this process involves the epidermis only).

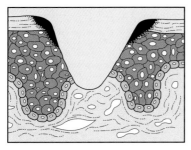

3 Ulcer (this affects both the dermis and epidermis).

The natural history of a cutaneous ulcer of any cause depends on many factors, including secondary infection, the patient's underlying immune status, systemic disorders, and dermatologic diseases – and that is just to mention a few. In addition, the patient's history may be inaccurate. She may be unaware of how long an ulcer has been present, or whether any significant changes have occurred.

A biopsy is an important diagnostic test, especially for a chronic ulcer. The biopsy should be taken from the edge of the lesion rather than from its base. A wedge excision from normal skin to the ulcer base will provide the best information for the pathologist. If this is impractical, two or more punch biopsies, from opposite sides of the lesion, should be considered. Some infections may be recognized in biopsy tissue, but appropriate cultures should always be obtained before beginning therapy. With acute ulcers, a biopsy may not be necessary if bacterial, viral, and/or fungal cultures are performed promptly to establish the diagnosis before beginning treatment.

The most serious diagnostic error is to guess at the etiology of an ulcer and to treat it empirically before all the data have been gathered. This error is usually made when a vulvar ulcer is erroneously assumed to be a sexually transmitted disease. In general, non-infectious vulvar ulcers are due to primary dermatologic diseases, but secondary infection can occur in open lesions. Bacterial and candidal infections should be treated, but it should not be assumed that they are the primary cause of chronic ulcers.

TABLE 1 DIFFERENTIAL DIAGNOSIS OF VULVAR ULCERS[1].

Figure	Cause	DIAGNOSIS	DIAGNOSTIC TEST	ASSOCIATED FINDINGS
Solitary ulcer (usually)				
4	○	Chancroid	Culture	*Haemophilus ducreyi*
5	○	Syphilis	Darkfield	*Treponema pallidum*
6	●	Pyoderma gangrenosum	Biopsy	Systemic disease: myeloma, bowel disease
7	●	Basal cell carcinoma	Biopsy	Localized pearly translucent borders with telangiectasia
8	●	Squamous cell carcinoma	Biopsy	Human papillomavirus (HPV), lichen sclerosus, other chronic inflammation or scarring processes
Multiple ulcers				
9	○	Herpes simplex, primary	Viral culture	Herpes simplex virus (HSV),
10	○	Herpes simplex, recurrent	Viral culture	HSV
11	○	Syphilis	Darkfield	*T. pallidum*
12	○	Varicella-zoster	Viral culture	Varicella-zoster virus, unilateral distribution
13	○	Candidiasis	Fungal culture	*Candida albicans* (*C. glabrata, C. paropsilosis,* and others)
14	●	Trauma: excoriation, factitia	None	Linear excoriations, lichenification
15	●	Behçet's syndrome	Biopsy	Constellation of arthritis, uveitis, other signs
16	●	Aphthosis	Biopsy	Lesions recurrent, often occur in mouth also
Granulomatous (heaped up)				
17	○	Syphilis (condylomata lata)	Darkfield, serology	Rising titer in serum, often generalized lesions
18	○	Granuloma inguinale (donovanosis)	Biopsy, special stains	*Calymmatobacterium granulomatis*
19	○	Lymphogranuloma venereum	Serum antigen tests	*Chlamydia trachomatis (serotypes L1, L2, L3)*
20	○	Diaper granulomas	Fungal culture	*Candida* spp.
21	●	Hidradenitis suppurativa	Biopsy	Are there axillary lesions? Lack of bowel disease
22	●	Crohn's (ulcerative colitis)	Biopsy	Bowel disease
23	●	Lymphangiectasis	Biopsy	History of chronic vulvar edema. Rule out HPV
24	●	Vulvar intraepithelial neoplasia (VIN)	Biopsy	History of cervical dysplasia, infection with HPV
25	●	Leukemia or lymphoma	Biopsy	Other lesions on body

Figure	Cause	DIAGNOSIS	DIAGNOSTIC TEST	ASSOCIATED FINDINGS
Recurrent ulcers*				
10	○	Herpes simplex	Viral culture	HSV, recurrent
13	○	Candidiasis	Fungal culture	*C. albicans (C. glabrata, C. paropsilosis,* and others)
15	●	Behçet's syndrome	Biopsy	Constellation of arthritis, uveitis, other signs
16	●	Aphthosis	Biopsy	Lesions recurrent, often occur in mouth also

* Erosive dermatoses may seem recurrent as they tend to flare and remit – see below.

Figure	Cause	DIAGNOSIS	DIAGNOSTIC TEST	ASSOCIATED FINDINGS
Erosive (superficial)				
26	○	Inflammatory vaginitis	Wet prep., culture	*Trichomonas* spp., *Gardnerella* spp.
27	○	Candidiasis	KOH prep., culture	*Candida* spp., satellite pustules on skin
28	○	Impetigo (*Staphylococcus* spp.)	Culture	Follicular pustules, peeling
30	●	Lichen planus	Biopsy	Erosive mucosa, including oral mucous membranes
31	●	Lichen sclerosus	Biopsy	Not on mucosa, loss of vulvar architecture
32	●	Plasma cell vulvitis	Biopsy	Etiology not known, may be asymptomatic
33	●	Fixed drug eruption	Biopsy	Ingestion of tetracycline, laxatives, other drugs
34	●	Necrolytic migratory erythema (glucagonoma)	Alpha-cell pancreatic tumor	Periorificial and intertriginous dermatitis; resolves when tumor is resected
29	○	Extramammary Paget's disease	Biopsy	Usually perianal, asymptomatic, chronic

Figure	Cause	DIAGNOSIS	DIAGNOSTIC TEST	ASSOCIATED FINDINGS
Blisters and erosions				
35	●	Contact dermatitis	Biopsy, patch testing	Often due to neomycin, latex, preservatives in topical agents, perfumes
36	●	Erythema multiforme	Biopsy	Target lesions, especially palms and soles, mucous membranes; associated with HSV, drugs
37		*Bullous pemphigoid*		Immunoglobulin G and C3 at dermoepidermal junction
38		*Pemphigus*		Immunoglobulin G between epidermal cells
		Dermatitis herpetiformis		Immunoglobulin A in papillary dermis
39		*Benign familial pemphigus (Hailey-Hailey disease)*		Negative immunoglobulin

[1] ○ = Infectious; ● = Non-infectious; ● = Malignant.

Color code for box outlines on the following pages

▢ = Infectious ▢ = Non-infectious ▢ = Malignant.

SOLITARY ULCERS

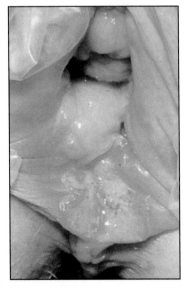

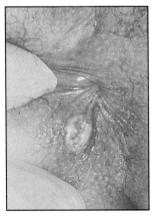

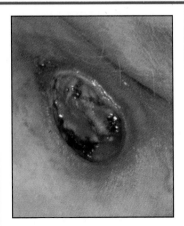

4 Chancroid. Painful superficial ulcers may be seen in this sexually transmitted disease caused by *Haemophilus ducreyi*. Multiple lesions are usually contiguous, giving the appearance of a large irregular erosion with a granulomatous base. About 50% of affected women have inguinal adenopathy.

5 Syphilis. Primary syphilitic chancre is a painless button-like lesion, with a central shallow ulceration. Multiple lesions can occur, especially in immunocompromised patients. Serum tests are usually not positive while the primary chancre is present.

6 Pyoderma gangrenosum. The lesion of pyoderma gangrenosum is a deep necrotic ulcer with dusky overhanging borders. It is not infectious, and may occur in patients with various systemic diseases, especially inflammatory bowel disease.

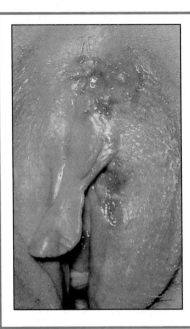

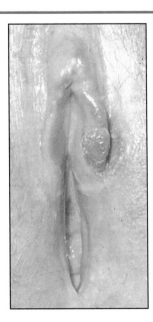

7 Basal cell carcinoma. The 'rodent ulcer', with its pearly telangiectatic border and necrotic center, is usually found on sun-exposed skin, though 10% of these lesions occur on covered portions of the body. Basal cell carcinomas rarely metastasize, but local invasion can cause significant tissue destruction.

8 Squamous cell carcinoma. Erosive or nodular lesions are often associated with chronic inflammation or scarring, such as in this patient with lichen sclerosus. In this case, carcinoma was found in the groin lymph nodes.

MULTIPLE ULCERS

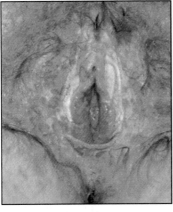

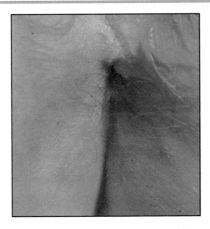

10 Herpes simplex virus (HSV). This condition is seen often because it recurs often. Blisters are often rubbed off by vulvar skin folds, forming shallow erosions. HSV may also recur as a solitary painful papule, resembling a 'pimple' or 'hair bump'. If present, the prodromal discomfort is a helpful diagnostic clue, and lesions are very tender until they heal. (They are also infectious until they heal.)

9 Primary herpes simplex virus (HSV). Primary HSV infections tend to be widespread and painful. Recurrences are usually localized and occur in variable sites within the area of the primary eruption.

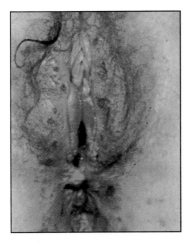

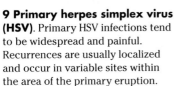

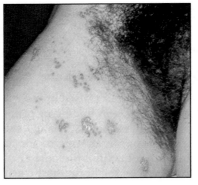

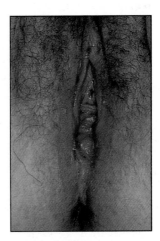

12 Varicella-zoster (shingles). Groups of umbilicated vesicles localized to a dermatome are typical of herpes zoster; herpes simplex virus (HSV) is usually a single group of vesicles. Zoster is unlikely to recur; HSV typically recurs. Immuno-compromised patients are more likely to develop both types of herpes infections; zoster may generalize to the entire body and HSV may become a large indolent ulcer. Treatment with acyclovir requires a four-fold dose increase for zoster, so it is important to differentiate the two conditions.

11 Syphilis (condylomata lata). Secondary syphilitic lesions typically generalize, particularly on the palms and soles. Genital plaques (condylomata lata) may resemble genital warts (condylomata acuminata). Lesions may ulcerate on mucous membranes (mucous patches). Serum tests for syphilis are strongly positive at this stage; moist lesions are highly contagious.

13 Candidiasis. Vaginal candidiasis is common, and lesions often spread to the vulva. Peeling and erosions are seen in intertriginous areas, and satellite pustules are scattered at the periphery. In contrast, tinea infections do not have satellite lesions; tiny vesiculopustules occur along the lesional border.

MULTIPLE ULCERS

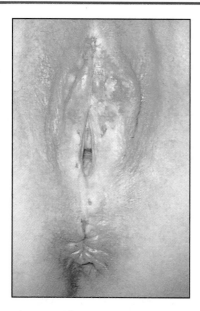

14 Trauma – excoriation or factitia. Leathery thickening of the skin (lichenification) is a result of chronic scratching (pruritus vulvae). The top layer becomes scaly and white, but vulvar anatomy is preserved, unlike the loss of architecture which results from lichen sclerosus. Shallow erosions due to the patient's scratching are called excoriations. In some cases, ulcers may be self-induced (factitial) by a variety of means.

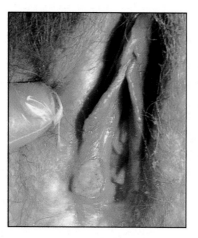

15 Behçet's syndrome. A relatively rare disorder, Behçet's syndrome is a complex multisystem disease. For a positive diagnosis, oral aphthae must be present, with at least two of the following: genital aphthae, synovitis, arthritis, cutaneous pustular vasculitis, posterior uveitis (retinal vasculitis), or meningoencephalitis. The absence of inflammatory bowel disease and collagen vascular diseases must be documented. Lesions tend to be deep and may scar. Flares and remissions are typical.

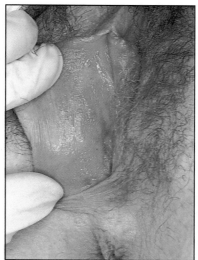

16 Aphthosis (canker sores). Patients with complex aphthosis have recurrent oral and genital aphthae which tend to be more frequent and more superficial than those of Behçet's syndrome. No other features of Behçet's syndrome can be identified. Treatment of early lesions with potent topical steroids can be very effective.

GRANULOMATOUS (HEAPED-UP) LESIONS

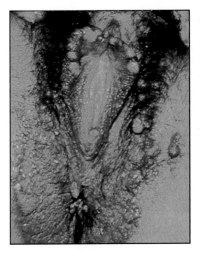

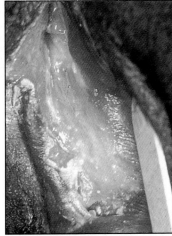

18 Granuloma inguinale (donovanosis). Necrotizing ulcerations in anogenital areas may be obscured by edema of the labia majora, as seen here. Early lesions are small eroded papules, which progress to hypertrophic, velvety, beefy-red, granulation tissue. Inguinal adenopathy does not occur unless secondary infection is present.

17 Syphilis (condylomata lata). Condylomata lata are papular lesions of secondary syphilis found in intertriginous areas where rubbing and maceration occur. The surface of the lesion is flat, clean, and moist; darkfield examination reveals swarms of treponemes. These are the most infectious lesions of syphilis.

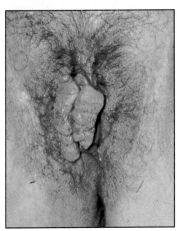

19 Lymphogranuloma venereum (LGV). Although ulcers are not typical of LGV, the diagnosis should be considered when edema of the labia is a prominent feature. The condition is most prevalent in tropical and subtropical areas, and usually presents with unilateral or bilateral enlargement of inguinal lymph nodes (buboes), which may mat together above and below the inguinal ligament (groove sign). Vulvar edema (elephantiasis) is known as esthiomène.

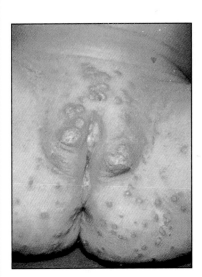

20 Diaper granuloma (granuloma gluteale infantum). These benign reddish-brown granulomatous nodules appear to be a cutaneous response to local inflammation, maceration, and secondary infection, usually with *Candida albicans*. They may resemble condylomata lata of syphilis, Kaposi's sarcoma, or lymphomas. Biopsy is helpful. Lesions of granuloma gluteale infantum resolve completely and spontaneously, within several months after treatment of the inflammation and secondary infection.

GRANULOMATOUS (HEAPED-UP) LESIONS

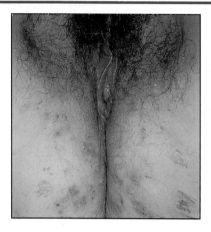

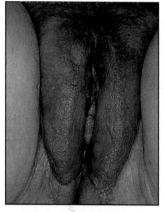

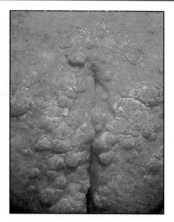

21 Hidradenitis suppurativa.
Comedones, furuncles, sinus tracts, and scars are typical of hidradenitis suppurativa. Like cystic acne, this is a chronic scarring disease of the apocrine glands that occurs in the axillae and groin. Mild cases can be controlled with antibiotics, such as minocycline or trimethoprim-sulfamethoxazole (depending on which organisms are predominant). Oral retinoids, which have been so successful for facial acne, have been disappointing for hidradenitis. For severe cases, excision and grafting of the involved tissue is usually the treatment of choice.

22 Crohn's disease, ulcerative colitis.
Granulomatous nodules can give a cobblestone appearance to the mucosa in patients with Crohn's disease. A diffuse granulomatous thickening of the labia has also been reported in early inflammatory bowel disease. Rectal fissures and fistulae are often present, and deep 'knife-cut' ulcerations can occur in the inguinal folds.

23 Lymphangiectasis. In patients with chronic vulvar edema, dilation of the lymphatic vessels can result in a verrucous surface, which can be difficult to distinguish from infection with human papillomavirus. In this case, the edema was due to chronic radiation dermatitis.

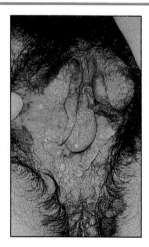

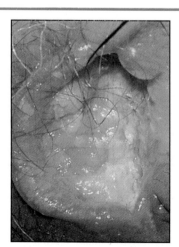

24 Vulvar intraepithelial neoplasia (VIN).
Scaly, erythematous papules and plaques are typical of squamous cell carcinoma *in situ* or VIN. Biopsies should be taken from the thickest parts of the lesion(s) and several areas should be sampled, as VIN is typically multifocal.

25 Leukemia, lymphoma.
Cutaneous infiltrates are not uncommon in lymphomas; this is a case of chronic myeloid leukemia. Biopsy should be performed for diagnosis. Cutaneous lesions may ulcerate during chemotherapy.

SUPERFICIAL EROSIONS

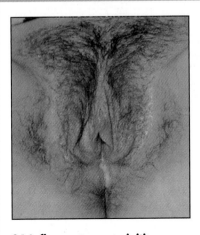

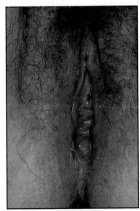

27 Candidiasis. Vaginal candidiasis is common, and lesions often spread to the vulva. Peeling and erosions are seen in intertriginous areas, and satellite pustules are scattered at the periphery. In contrast, tinea infections do not have satellite lesions; tiny vesiculopustules occur along the lesional border.

26 Inflammatory vaginitis. Although vulvar edema and inflammation is most often associated with candidal vulvovaginitis, other causes should also be considered. This is an example of trichomoniasis. Contact or irritant dermatitis to vaginal medication is another possibility.

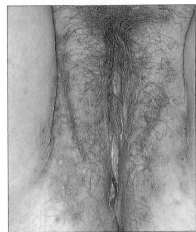

28 Impetigo (*Staphylococcus* spp.). Staphylococcal infection of the skin begins as follicular pustules, then spreads as thin-walled bullae that soon erode, leaving a moist superficial surface with peeling edges. Vulvar and perineal impetigo is particularly common in human immunodeficiency virus (HIV) infection and acquired immunodeficiency syndrome (AIDS).

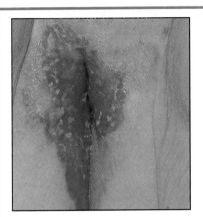

29 Extramammary Paget's disease. Diagnosis of this lesion depends on the examiner's index of suspicion and a biopsy. As it resembles a dermatitis and grows slowly, it is not usually recognized for one to two years. It may be associated with an underlying apocrine, eccrine, or adenoid carcinoma.

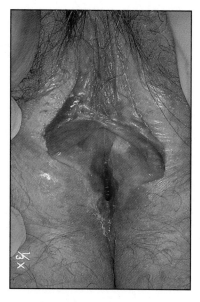

30 Lichen planus (LP). Erosions of LP are often limited to vaginal and introital mucosae. It is helpful to examine the gums and oral mucosa, since LP often affects both areas. Lesions are chronic and recurrent.

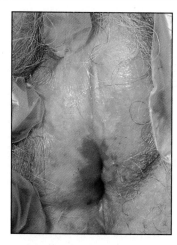

31 Lichen sclerosus (LS). In general, this is not as likely to erode spontaneously as LP. When the epithelium is damaged, it is usually the result of excoriation by the patient. In this case, a traumatic fissure in the posterior introitus has become secondarily infected with *Candida*. The diagnosis of LS was made by a biopsy of the whitened epithelium on the perineum.

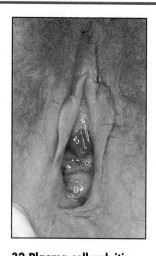

32 Plasma cell vulvitis. This bright red eruption (also called vulvitis circumscripta plasmacellularis) is limited to the mucous membranes and may be asymptomatic, though patients usually complain of tenderness. Lesions resolve slowly, leaving a rusty 'stain' on the skin as they disappear. Recurrences are common, and the etiology is not known. (A similar eruption may occur on the male glans penis, where it is known as Zoon's balanitis.)

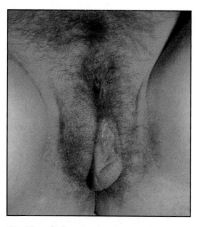

33 Fixed drug eruption. The erosion on the edematous labium minus will recur each time the patient ingests the medication responsible – in this case, a combination of sulfamethoxazole and trimethoprim. Other areas on the body may also be affected, but the localized round, macular eruption does not involve the entire skin. When lesions resolve, the skin is often left hyperpigmented. Tetracycline and phenolphthalein are common offending agents.

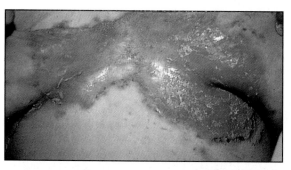

34 Necrolytic migratory erythema (glucagonoma). This unusual eruption typically involves the intertriginous areas, such as the inframammary folds (shown here), the axillae, and the groin. Lesions also occur around the mouth and the anus, as well as on the extremities. The patient has an alpha-cell tumor of the pancreas (glucagonoma) and serum levels of glucagon are markedly elevated. Provided the examiner is familiar with this paraneoplastic syndrome, the eruption's peculiar nature is sufficiently characteristic to make the diagnosis possible.

BLISTERS AND EROSIONS

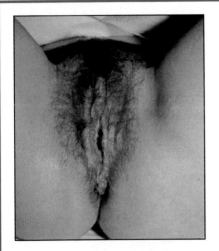

35 Contact dermatitis. Contact or irritant dermatitis may be caused by a medication or cleaning agent used by the patient because of an underlying problem, so infection should be considered in the overall evaluation. An irritant reaction typically causes immediate burning and stinging, usually because the agent has been applied to inflamed skin. A contact allergen does not initiate a dermatitis until about two days after application; the eruption lasts two to three weeks.

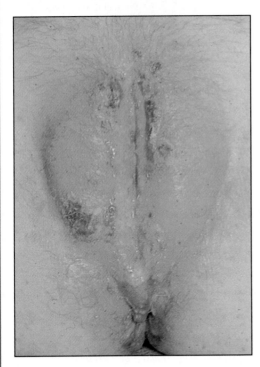

36 Erythema multiforme (Stevens–Johnson syndrome). Erythema multiforme (EM) is a cutaneous reaction pattern recognized in its early stages by target-shaped lesions on the palms and soles, as well as on the rest of the body. The most common causes are Mycoplasma pneumoniae, recurrent herpes simplex virus (HSV), in which EM follows each HSV outbreak, and various drugs. However, many cases are idiopathic.

BLISTERS AND EROSIONS

IMMUNOLOGIC BULLAE

The immunologically mediated cutaneous blistering diseases have been extensively studied. Biopsies for routine histopathology and immunofluorescent staining are recommended (the latter requires a special fixative). Lesions are rarely limited to the genitalia, and systemic immunosuppressive therapy is usually necessary.

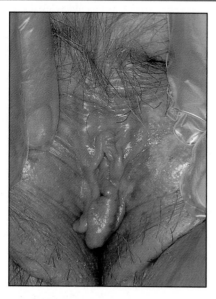

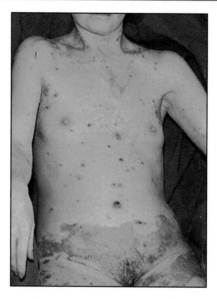

37 Bullous pemphigoid. This usually occurs in older patients and typically has large tense bullae. Immunoglobulin is deposited along the basement membrane. A somewhat rare form is cicatricial pemphigoid, which affects mucous membranes and causes scarring – eye lesions can cause blindness.

38 Pemphigus. This usually presents with thin-walled blisters, which are easily traumatized, leaving erosions. The immunoglobulins are deposited between epithelial cells, causing them to lose their adherence to one another.

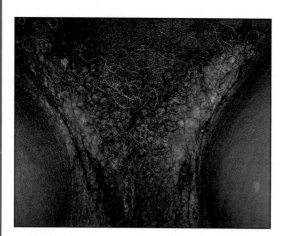

39 Benign familial pemphigus. This is a chronic and recurrent eruption of the axillae and groin; it usually occurs in several family members and has an equal predilection for males and females. The diagnosis is confirmed by an absence of immunoglobulins and the histopathology.

Appendix B

Topical Steroids in the Therapy of Vulvar Diseases

Marilynne McKay

Just as the obstetrician-gynecologist develops facility with the use of oral estrogen-containing preparations, the dermatologist must learn to choose the best topical steroid preparation for the patient and her problem. It is no more appropriate to ask a dermatologist for the "best steroid" than it would be to ask a gynecologist for the "best estrogen." The answer always depends on many considerations, such as the condition being treated, the patient's age and reliability, the length of time the medication will be used, and the potential side effects.

Like oral estrogen preparations, some generalizations can be made about topical steroids:

• There are more kinds than you really need.
• The strongest isn't necessarily the best.
• Side effects are often the limiting factor.
• The patient's preference may determine which medication you choose.
• They won't work if not used as directed.

Unlike drug combinations with oral estrogens, combinations of topical steroids with other drugs have not been as effective as might be expected. A well-known combination of a potent topical steroid (betamethasone dipropionate) and an antifungal (clotrimazole) has been responsible for numerous instances of steroid rebound dermatitis and can even cause striae formation with prolonged use. For some reason, the antifungal does not seem to be as effective in this combination form either. The best advice is to learn to use a few topical steroids well and know which conditions to treat with them.

CHOOSING A TOPICAL STEROID: POTENCY AND VEHICLES

Topical steroids are grouped into classes (I-VII) based on their potency as measured by a standardized vasoconstrictor assay. Simply stated, this test measures how long blanching persists on the forearm after a measured amount of a steroid is applied. The longer blanching (vasoconstriction) persists, the more potent the steroid. Note that fluorination has nothing to do with the potency classification. The higher the potency, the more side effects, whether the corticosteroid is fluorinated or not. (When topical steroids were first developed, fluorination was linked to potency, but this is no longer a hard-and-fast rule.)

Class VII topical steroids are relatively safe and are now available in the United States without a prescription. They are effective anti-inflammatory and emollient agents, are safe to use in intertriginous areas (axillae and groin) as well as the face, and have a low risk of candida superinfection. For patients with chronic dermatitis (e.g., atopy) the Class VII steroids can prevent flares which might occur if steroids were discontinued altogether.

Class IV mid-potency topical steroids are actually "full strength" medications which have been the dermatologic standard for years. Because vulvar skin absorbs steroids well (and is also an occluded area), these are the highest strength needed for most vulvar problems. They are considerably safer than the high-potency preparations, but still have significant side effects, so must be prescribed in judicious amounts.

Class I "Superpotent" topical steroids are remarkable medications[1,2]. Regular applications are equivalent to intralesional injections, but it is difficult to control the area treated. On the vulva, where several skin surfaces are in contact with one another, this can be a problem. There is significant systemic absorption with the Class I steroids: studies have shown that 2 grams (the size of a sample tube) per day of 0.05% clobetasol propionate can suppress the hypothalamic–pituitary–adrenal axis[3,4]. It has been recommended that usage of clobetasol propionate 0.05% (Dermovate, Temovate) should not exceed 50gm/week[5]; this is approximately the size of a large prescription tube. The dosage should be tapered as soon as improvement is noted and should be discontinued after two weeks if there is no response. Class I steroids should not be prescribed for children under the age of 12[6]. Medicolegal precedent in the U.K. and U.S.A. has linked long-term Class I steroid usage with aseptic necrosis of the femoral head[7], glaucoma and cataracts[8], and extensive irreversible striae formation.

COMPLICATIONS

In addition to the systemic effects described above, there are a number of local complications. Striae are particularly likely to occur on the thin skin of the inner thighs and abdomen, and topical steroids applied to the vulva almost invariably affect these areas due to anatomical contact. Bruising or petechial (non-blanching) erythema are the first signs of steroid side-effects.

After use for more than six weeks, topical steroids with potencies of Class V or higher can cause steroid rebound dermatitis to one degree or another when they are discontinued. Loss of steroid vaso-constriction results in rebound vasodilation of the cutaneous capillaries, often with burning discomfort which can only be relieved with re-application of the topical steroid. The likelihood of this complication increases with the potency of the preparation, and patients who are rosacea-prone (those with fair skin and a tendency to flush easily) are particularly susceptible, whether the steroid is applied to the face or to the vulva.

Local immunosuppression of vulvar skin with high-potency steroids may also potentiate acute outbreaks of recurrent herpes simplex and human papillo-mavirus. Concomitant therapy with topical steroids may also increase or sustain the severity of infections (candidiasis, tinea, staphylococcus) and infestations such as scabies[9].

CREAM OR OINTMENT?

Potency depends on the vehicle in which the steroid is mixed. Vehicles must carry the drug through the skin: a difficult task, since a major function of the stratum corneum is to be a barrier to outside agents. Much research goes into developing vehicles which will be non-irritating, cosmetically elegant, and effec-tive in maximizing delivery of the steroid to the dermis.

The basic principle is that when the stratum corneum is hydrated, medications penetrate better. This is why creams are so effective: as mixtures of water and oil, they hydrate the skin with water and "seal in" the moisture with oil. Occlusion keeps the skin moist by retarding evaporation of water, so ointment bases (like petroleum jelly) which are more occlusive allow medications to penetrate for a longer time, especially when they are applied to moist skin immediately after a bath.

Ointment-based steroids are more potent than the same preparation in a cream or lotion base because ointments are more occlusive. Another advantage to ointments is that they are less likely to contain allergens like preservatives, which are necessary in water-based creams. Unfortunately, many patients don't care for the "greasy" feel of ointments, so they don't use them as often as they should. Gels also penetrate well, usually because they contain propy-lene glycol, a good vehicle for carrying drugs through the skin. Propylene glycol can be irritating, however, and patients with irritated mucosal surfaces (vulvar inflammation) often complain of stinging with gels.

Special "optimized" vehicles can increase the potency of a preparation by one or even two classes, even though the concentration of drug is the same. This is how pharmaceutical companies constantly jockey for position on the steroid potency chart, and why generic preparations are an unknown quantity. Some generic creams or ointments are be significantly less effective because the vehicle does not deliver the drug as well as expected. There is no good way to predict this except by experience, because only brand-name drugs are included in the "relative potency" evaluation. (Dermatologists who use these medications more frequently may have better experience with generic preparations, but many of them prefer specific brands because they are more predictable.) Mixing one's own steroid preparations is discouraged — these are even more unreliable than generic brands.

WHEN NOT TO USE HIGH-POTENCY STEROIDS

Two questions should be asked when choosing a steroid: "What am I treating?" and "How long should it take to bring the condition under control?" If you are unsure about either (or both!) of these, then you should NOT prescribe a Class I or II high-potency preparation. The patient is likely to develop side effects if a Class I or II steroid is applied for too long a time. Likewise, if the steroid is not used long enough for an appropriate treatment trial, there will be minimal benefit and it will be unclear if the medication has been effective. Don't use Class I or II topicals for erythema alone, vulvodynia (burning) or itching in the absence of skin disease, or for histopathology of non-diagnostic mild squamous cell hyperplasia.

OTHER TOPICAL MEDICATIONS

Burow's Solution compresses

For open, oozing dermatitis, Burow's solution (aluminum acetate) is an excellent astringent and antiseptic. It is somewhat anesthetic as well, and is particularly effective in treating primary herpes simplex infections. Tablets or powder packets may be obtained at the pharmacy; one packet dissolved in one pint of water makes a 1:40 solution, which is recommended for topical application. The patient should mix the solution fresh daily, but it can be used throughout the day. A washcloth or soft gauze should be saturated with the solution and applied to the vulva and left in place for 20 minutes three or four times daily. The patient may sit on a folded towel to absorb excess moisture, or may find it more convenient to sit in a dry bathtub. The compress should be kept moist and not allowed to dry; rinsing is not necessary.

Sea water sitz baths

The main benefit of this preparation over self-mixed salt solution is the relatively constant concentration of ingredients; in addition to sodium chloride, magnesium sulfate and other salts are also included. Packets of powdered salts may be found where aquarium supplies are sold, and mixing instructions are usually by the gallon. This makes preparation of a sitz bath more convenient, and this solution has been recommended for pain relief and healing after laser or electrosurgical procedures.

Topical acyclovir ointment

Although this medication has been shown to decrease viral shedding when used in combination with oral acyclovir in primary herpes simplex (HSV) infections, it has not been proven efficacious in recurrent HSV. Oral acyclovir is effective in recurrent HSV and may be taken on a daily basis to suppress HSV outbreaks. There does not, however, appear to be any justification in the use of topical acyclovir ointment as a therapeutic agent in recurrent HSV.

Eurax-Valisone cream

Eurax (crotamiton) is a scabicide and antipruritic cream that is not as effective for scabies as lindane (Kwell) or permethrin (Elimite). The antipruritic effect is achieved by mild skin irritation which distracts from the sensation of "itch." The late vulvologist, Dr. Eduard G. Friedrich, Jr., recommended mixing 3 parts Eurax with 7 parts betamethasone valerate 0.1% cream (Valisone) for pruritic vulvar dermatoses. The reasoning for this mixture was that the antipruritic effect of the crotamiton would provide immediate relief of itching while the topical Class V steroid would gradually treat the underlying skin condition. There are two problems with this mixture: (1) crotamiton is an irritant, and causes marked stinging on skin which is already inflamed; (2) a mixture is significantly more expensive than two tubes of medication. There is nothing particularly "scientific" about the 3:7 mixture; equal parts could be used for intense pruritus and the steroid could be

tapered gradually in favor of the crotamiton for persistent or occasional itch. The topical steroid is the most important ingredient and it should be prescribed as noted below. Crotamiton may be considered an "anti-itch" cream which the patient may apply whenever she wishes — but it should only be used on thickened, scaly lesions where pruritus is the major complaint.

Topical testosterone ointment

2% testosterone propionate in petrolatum was long considered the mainstay of treatment for lichen sclerosus. Topical testosterone was never recommended for vulvar dermatoses other than lichen sclerosus, although it was widely used as a "treatment trial" when gynecologists were unsure why patients had symptomatic vulvar itching or burning. It was thought that the androgenic effect served somehow to "toughen" vulvar skin in opposition to influences of estrogen. This has not been found to be the case; improvement with topical testosterone has probably been due to the conversion of androgenic steroid to glucocorticoid within the skin itself. Testosterone ointment has not been found to be as effective as topical steroids for vulvar dermatoses, and new data has shown the Class I steroids to be more effective in the treatment of lichen sclerosus[10, 11,12]. Side effects of topical testosterone include clitoral hypertrophy, increased libido, local hair growth, deepening of the voice and other signs of masculinization which patients often find unpleasant.

HOW MUCH TO PRESCRIBE

30 grams is about one ounce. In the U.S. topical medications are dispensed by the ounce, so multiples of 30 are common (along with 15 gm and 45 gm tubes.) 60 grams (2 oz) will cover the whole body twice. A 30-gm tube of cream, rubbed in well, will be enough for a patient to apply to the entire vulva three times daily for a week. (Applying medication more than that is probably wasting it. Twice daily is generally enough, and tapering to once daily or every-other-day is a good way to decrease usage as the patient improves.) Patients sometimes think they have to re-apply creams to the entire vulva each time they wipe after using the commode, but this is not necessary. If a medication has been rubbed in well, it will be absorbed in about 30 minutes to the point that re-application is not necessary.

It is important to explain to the patient how much medication to use. Patients who expect a medication to stop the sensation of itching, for instance, may apply a thick layer of cream several times a day and protest that "it's not working" when she is still itching a week later (see below.) Patients who are concerned about the cost of medication may not use enough cream to treat the condition. Always ask how much cream ("how many tubes?") the patient has used since the last visit and counsel her accordingly. The patient information sheets following this appendix are helpful for specific disorders.

SUMMARY

Review the actual cost to the patient of topical steroids. While money can be saved by prescribing generic preparations, some of these aren't nearly as effective because the vehicle isn't as good at delivering the drug. (See Table of brand names and variations in potency between cream, oin tment, and optimized cream.) Choose an ointment-based steroid in Class I or II to use as a "strong medicine" (write that on the prescription so it will appear on the label that the patient will see — don't count on her to remember which cream is the most potent.) An ointment base is less pleasant to use, so a high-potency ointment will be more likely to be put aside in favor of a lower-potency Class IV "maintenance cream" (also written to appear on the prescription label). If a patient tells you that a topical is irritating, make a note of it. If you hear it from several patients, quit using it and choose another. Ointments and water-based creams are usually well-tolerated on the vulva.

Don't write unlimited refills or refill these by telephone. A flare of symptoms may be superinfection with Candida or recurrence of herpes simplex because of steroid immunosuppression. Steroid rebound dermatitis may cause the patient to use the topical steroid well beyond the time it should have been discontinued.

Skin problems take time to resolve, and the physician should counsel the patient accordingly. Patients are often confused about causes and effects of genital symptoms; they don't understand that damaged skin may itch or burn until it heals. They demand "tests to find out why I have this," and expect relief within a few days. This confusion may be worsened when the provider doesn't realize that symptomatic dermatoses typically take weeks to resolve. Changing prescriptions after only a few days makes the patient think that whatever disease she has can't be treated. Often the best therapy is persistent use of bland emollients or mild topical steroids and gentle but firm reassurance that no infection or malignancy has been discovered. With skin conditions, successful treatment gradually results in symptom improvement as therapy is continued, so treatment protocols should be continued for a fair trial of six to eight weeks.

HOW STEROIDS WORK
- Reduce inflammation
- Constrict cutaneous capillaries, directly decreasing erythema.
- Decrease the mitotic rate of rapidly proliferating epidermis
- Decrease fibroblast proliferation

STEROID SIDE EFFECTS WITH NORMAL USE
- Epidermal atrophy
- Dermal atrophy and striae formation
- Easy bruising
- Telangiectasias
- Steroid rebound dermatitis when discontinued

SYSTEMIC COMPLICATIONS OF CLASS I STEROIDS
- Suppression of hypothalamic–pituitary–adrenal axis
- Aseptic necrosis of the femoral head
- extensive irreversible striae formation
- glaucoma and cataracts (with facial application)

STEROID POTENCY DEPENDS ON
- corticosteroid formula
- concentration of steroid
- vehicle
- frequency of application and length of time used

STEROID-RESPONSIVE VULVAR DERMATOSES
- Thick, scaly lesions (usually pruritic)
  Lichen Sclerosus (LS)
  Psoriasis
  Lichen Simplex Chronicus (LSC)
- Blisters and erosions
  Lichen Planus (LP)
  Dermatitis/Eczema
  Bullous diseases

REMEMBER:
- Topical steroids are not a "cure."
- Use the lowest steroid potency that will control the problem.
- Chronic skin diseases require long-term therapy.
- Topical steroids can potentiate co-infections with candida, tinea, bacteria, and scabies.

Table 1 Topical Steroids in the Therapy of Vulvar Diseases

STEROID POTENCY*	CONDITION	ACTION OF STEROID	BENEFIT	BEST DOSAGE	RISK IF NOT USED AS DIRECTED
Super potent	Lichen sclerosus et atrophicus (LS)	Decreases inflammation leading to sclerotic process, thins scale, reduces sclerosis	Decreases itching, resolves scale and sclerosis	Super potent once daily for 4–6 weeks, then decrease frequency and potency	Overthinning of skin, steroid rebound dermatitis (SRD) with burning, telangiectasia formation, gluteal and thigh striae, candida superinfection
Highly potent	Thick, scaly plaque (psoriasis, lichen planus, lichen simplex chronicus)	Decreases inflammation and mitotic rate, thins scale, reduces thickness	Decreases itching, resolves scale and thickness	Highly potent daily for 3–4 weeks, then decrease	1) Patient may become resistant to formulation (tachyphylaxis) 2) Continued use affects normal skin
Highly potent	Erosive dermatoses (erosive lichen planus, bullous diseases)	Reduces inflammation; suppresses immune-mediated process causing blister formation	Reduces blister formation; re-epithelializes erosions	Highly potent cream or ointment; begin daily, then decrease	Secondary candida infection of erosions, delayed healing when blisters controlled, telangiectasias, SRD, striae on buttocks, thighs
Potent	Acute local cutaneous inflammation (allergic, irritant, atopic eczema or dermatitis), oozy wet	Vasoconstriction, reduces inflammation	Resolves inflammation, controls dermatitis, prevents blisters	Potent for flare, moderately potent for maintenance	Skin atrophy and fragility, easy bruising, secondary infection (bacteria, candida, fungi), telangiectasia, depigmentation
Moderately potent	Symptomatic vulvar (or facial) skin with mild erythema but without scaling or plaques, may itch or burn	Vasoconstriction reduces inflammation	Reduction of erythema, resolution of rash	Moderately potent AVOID HIGHER POTENCIES	Steroid rebound dermatitis (SRD) and burning sensation when steroid discontinued; continued need for stronger preparations to control SRD; telangiectasia formation
Mild	Normal skin vulvodynia Patient complains of burn, sting, irritation, rawness; NO VISIBLE RASH	Skin blanching from vasoconstriction	NONE	NONE	Skin atrophy and fragility, telangiectasia, rebound vasodilation and inflammation, secondary infection (bacteria, candida, fungi), bruising, depigmentation

* In the US:
High to moderate potency = Class I–III
Moderate to mild potency = Class IV–VII

Table 2 Topical Steroid Potency Ranking 1995

CLASS	GENERIC NAME	US BRAND NAME	UK BRAND NAME	FRANCE	ITALY	GERMANY	SPAIN
Super potent	Clobetasol propionate Betamethasone dipropionate Diflorasone diacetate Halobetasol propionate	Temovate, oint .05% Diprolene oint, AF cr .05% Psorcon oint .05% Ultravate cr, oint .05%	Dermovate cr, oint .05%	Dermaval	Clobetasol	Dermoxin	Clobate
Highly potent	Amcinonide Betamethasone dipropionate Desoximetasone Diflorasone diacetate Diflucortolone valerate Fluocinonide Halcinonide	Cyclocort cr, lot, oint .01% Diprosone, Maxivate cr, lot, oint .05% Topicort cr, oint, gel 0.25% Maxiflor, Florene cr, oint .05% Lidex cr, oint, gel, sol 0.1% Halog cr, oint, sol 0.1%	Diprosone cr, oint .05% Stiedex oily cream 0.25% Nerisone cr, oily cr, oint .01% Metosyn cr, oint .05% Halciderm cr .01%	Diprolene	Diprosone	Diprosone	Diproderm
Potent	Betamethasone valerate Beclomathasone dipropionate Desonide Fluocinolone acetonide Flurandrenolide Fluticasone propionate Hydrocortisone butyrate Hydrocortisone valerate Mometasone furoate Triamcinolone acetonide	Valisone cr, lotion, oint 0.1% Tridesilon oint .05% Synalar cr, oint .025%f Cordran cr, oint .05% Locoid cr, oint 0.1% Westcort cr, oint 0.2% Elocon cr, lotion, oint 0.1% Aristocort, Kenalog oint 0.1%	Betnovate cr, lotion, oint 0.1% Propaderm cr, oint .025% Synalar cr, oint .025% Cutivate cr .05% Locoid cr, oint 0.1% Elocon cr, oint 0.1% Adcortyl cr, oint 0.1%	Betnaval Synalar Kenacort-A	Ecoval-70 Propaderm Kanacort	Betnesol Volon-A	Betnovate Synalar
Moderately potent	Aclometasone dipropionate Clobetasone butyrate Desonide Flumethasone pivolate Fluocinolone acetonide Flurandrenolone Triamcinolone acetonide	Aclovate cr, oint .05% Tridesilon cr .05% Locorten cr .03% Synalar cr, sol .01% Aristocort, Kenalog cr, lot 0.1%, oint .025%	Modrasone cr, oint .05% Eumovate cr, oint .05% Haelan cr, oint .0125%	Aclosone	Legaderm Eumovate	Delonal Eumovate	Aclodal Eumovate
Mild	Hydrocortisone Hydrocortisone acetate	Cortdome, Eldecort, Dermacort, Hytone cr, oint, lot 1% & 2.5% Pramosone 1% & 2.5%	Dioderm, Efcortelan, Hydrocortisyl, Mildison cr, oint 1% Hydrocortistab cr, oint 1%	Hydrocortisone Astier	Algicortif Dermacoral	Hydrocortison e Wolff	Crema-Transcotanea-Asti

REFERENCES

1. Olsen EA, Cornell RC: Topical clobetasol-17-propionate: review of its clinical efficacy and safety. *J. Amer. Acad. Dermatol.* 1986;**15**: 246–55.
2. Harris DW, Hunter JA: The use and abuse of 0.05 per cent clobetasol propionate in dermatology. *Dermatol Clinics.* 1988; 6: 643–647.
3. Anonymous: Clobetasol proprionate (Temovate by Glaxo). *Drug Newslett* 1986; **5**(3):24.
4. Ohman EM, Rogers S, Meenan FO, et al: Adrenal suppression following low dose topical clobetasol propionate. *J. Roy. Soc. Med.* 1987; 80:422–423.
5. Carruthers JA, August PJ, Staughton RC: Observations on the systemic effect of topical clobetasol propionate (Dermovate). *B.M.J.* 1975; **4**(5990):203–204.
6. Stoppolini G: Potential hazards of topical steroid therapy. *Am J. Dis Child* 1983; **137**:1130–1131.
7. Hogan DJ, Sibley JT, Lane PR: Avascular necrosis of the hips following long-term use of clobetasol propionate. *J. Am. Acad. Dermatol.* 1986; **14**:515–517.
8. Katsushima H, Souma K, Nishio C, et al: Glaucoma and posterior subcapsular cataract after long-term use of corticosteroid lotion in a case with photodermatitis. *J. Clin. Ophthalmol.* 1986; 40:1345–1349.
9. Millard LG: Norwegian scabies developing during treatment with fluorinated steroid therapy. *Acta Dermato-Vener.* 1977; **57**(1):86–88.
10. Dalziel KL, Millard PR, Wojnarowska F. The treatment of vulval lichen sclerosus with a very potent topical steroid (clobetasol propionate 0.05%) cream. *Brit. J. Dermatol.* 1991; **124**:461–464.
11. Bracco GL, Carli P, Sonni L, *et al.* Clinical and histologic effects of topical treatments of vulval lichen sclerosus. A critical evaluation. *J Repro. Med.* 1993; **38**:37–40.
12. Cattaneo A, De Marco A, Sonni L, *et al.* Clobetasolo vs testosterone nel trattamento del lichen scleroso della regione vulvare. *Minerva Ginecologica.* 1992; **44**:567–571.

ACKNOWLEDGEMENTS
The following citations refer to the illustrations in Appendix A. Figures 4, 7, 14, 24, 25, are reproduced from V. R. Tindall. *Diagnostic picture tests in obstetrics and gynaecology.* London; Wolfe Medical Publications Ltd, 1981. Figures 8 and 36 are reproduced from V. R. Tindall. *Colour atlas of clinical gynaecology.* London; Wolfe Medical Publications Ltd, 1981. Figures 9, 10, 11, 12, 15, 17, 19, 20, 23, 26, 33, 35 are reproduced from A. Wisdom. *Colour atlas of sexually transmitted diseases.* London; Wolfe Medical Publications Ltd, 1989. Figure 38 is reproduced from G. M. Levene and S. K. Goolamali. *Diagnostic picture tests in dermatology.* London; Wolfe Medical Publications Ltd, 1986.

PATIENT INFORMATION – LICHEN PLANUS (*like-*in **plan-***us*)

Is lichen planus the same as "vulvar dystrophy"?

"Vulvar dystrophy" is an old name for several different skin conditions. Now we use a specific name (like *lichen planus*) whenever possible, because we have different treatments for each condition. By the way, there are other vulvar skin conditions with the word "lichen" in their name (lichen simplex, lichen sclerosus); these have NO relationship to lichen planus.

Lichen planus (LP) is a skin condition familiar to dermatologists. The usual form of this skin disorder is itchy bumps, especially on the shins, the inner wrists, and the hands. A rare type of lichen planus affects mucous membranes of the mouth and genitals. Both kinds of lichen planus can affect men and women, and patients often have both mouth and skin lesions. Vaginal lichen planus (also called "desquamative vaginitis" or erosive LP) isn't caused by vaginal infections, hormones, or aging. Skin with LP is moist and red (eroded) because the top layer rubs off very easily.

How is lichen planus diagnosed?

Lichen planus can resemble other vulvar skin disorders, but LP is the major one that involves the vagina as well as the vulva. Some blistering skin diseases (pemphigus, pemphigoid) also produce vulvar erosions. A biopsy is usually necessary to diagnose lichen planus. This is usually a minor procedure done in the office with a local anesthetic — removing a small plug of skin can answer many questions for you and your doctor.

How did I get lichen planus?

No one knows how lichen planus starts, but we don't think that it's because of anything you did or didn't do. Most patients just develop LP for no apparent reason. It is not an infection that you caught from anyone, and you certainly can't give it to anyone else. LP lesions result from inflammation in the skin, but we don't know what makes lesions develop in one place or another. The thin mucous membranes inside the mouth and vagina lose their top layer when they become inflamed, so red erosions rather than bumps develop when LP affects these areas.

What kinds of problems can I have with LP?

Lichen planus on the skin is often extremely itchy and it may be difficult to control lesions, even with high-potency medications. Erosive lichen planus can be painful in the mouth and vagina, and these areas can become infected. Vaginal erosions on opposing surfaces may "heal together" forming thin scar tissue that narrows the vagina. Surgical separation of these surfaces is relatively easy, however, and using vaginal dilators and cortisone creams can help prevent scar formation.

Can LP be treated? Is it curable?

Lichen planus is a skin condition, and usually improves with certain kinds of creams and ointments. Although the skin may not look entirely normal when it heals, medications control itching and erosion. In some cases, LP just seems to come and go on its own. The purpose of therapy is to decrease inflammation, and steroids seem to do this the best. When a disease is limited to the skin, creams and ointments are best, because of complications with steroids given by mouth. There is not presently any one ideal treatment for erosive LP, but several new drugs have been promising. Dermatologists generally know the most about new treatments for LP.

From Black, McKay & Braude: Color Atlas and Text of Obstetric and Gynecologic Dermatology, *Mosby–Wolfe, London 1995. © Times Mirror International Publishers Ltd.*

PATIENT INFORMATION – LICHEN PLANUS *continued*

If LP is not an infection, why do antibiotics help?

The top layer of the skin is a barrier against all kinds of bacteria. When this layer is lost, then the moist lower layers of skin can become infected. This secondary infection can keep the skin from healing as rapidly as it could — antibiotic vaginal creams and oral medications control germs that keep the skin from healing.

What role does yeast (Candida) play in LP?

Candida organisms grow very well in a moist environment where there is no skin barrier. They also thrive when steroids or antibiotics are used, and Candida infection can keep the skin from healing properly. Your doctor may have you use a vaginal or oral anti-candidal medication once or twice a week when you are being treated for a flare of symptoms.

Is there a chance that LP could turn into cancer?

Lichen planus scars the skin, and this is a risk for developing a local type of skin cancer. (This has been reported in men with LP on the penis more often than in women with vaginal LP.) The signs of a developing skin cancer are similar to those on other parts of the body: a sore or ulcer that doesn't heal in a few weeks, a lesion that continues to bleed easily, or a bump or raised lesion that is getting progressively larger. If these don't heal despite regular use of your prescribed medication, then let your doctor have a look. It may be that your cream or ointment needs to be changed, but a biopsy might be necessary to be certain that all is well.

What should I watch for?

Because LP is likely to flare and remit, you should pay close attention to vaginal discharge, which may indicate that erosion and/or secondary infection has developed. If you have had problems with vaginal narrowing, regular use of dilators may prevent this. Medication should be used on a regular maintenance basis, rather than only for severe flares, which are much harder to bring under control. You should have regular (at least yearly) visits to a gynecologist or dermatologist who knows about lichen planus. This is not necessarily a "premalignant" condition, but your doctor should do a biopsy any time he or she thinks a change might be abnormal.

PATIENT INFORMATION – LICHEN SCLEROSUS (*like-in skler-o-sus*)

Is lichen sclerosus the same as "vulvar dystrophy"?

"Vulvar dystrophy" is an old name for several different skin conditions. Now we use a specific name (like lichen sclerosus) whenever possible, because we have different treatments for each condition. By the way, there are other vulvar skin conditions with the word "lichen" in their name (lichen simplex, lichen planus); these have NO relationship to lichen sclerosus.

Lichen sclerosus (LS) is a skin condition familiar to dermatologists and gynecologists. It can affect men, women, or children, but is more common in women. The cause is unknown, but it is not due to vaginal infections, menopause, or aging. Skin with LS loses color and becomes thin and fragile.

How did I get lichen sclerosus?

No one knows how lichen sclerosus starts, but we don't think that it's because of anything you did or didn't do. It is not an infection that you caught from anyone, and you certainly can't give it to anyone else. There have been a few reports of sisters or mothers and daughters with LS, so this may indicate a possible inherited tendency to develop this condition, but this is quite unusual. Most patients just develop LS by themselves for no apparent reason. Patients with LS sometimes have other diseases that have antibodies to the body's own tissue, like thyroid disease or diabetes. However, there is no evidence that this process causes LS itself. Patients with autoimmune diseases do not seem to be more likely to develop lichen sclerosus.

Why do I itch so much? Have I ruined my skin by scratching?

Patients with lichen sclerosus report very different degrees of discomfort. Some with only a few areas of LS have extreme itching or burning, while others with LS on the entire vulva have no symptoms at all. In other words, there does not seem to be a relation between severity of LS and symptoms. Even skin badly damaged by scratching will gradually heal when it is left alone.

Can LS be treated? Is it curable?

Lichen sclerosus is a skin condition, and improves with certain kinds of creams and ointments. Although the skin may not entirely return to its normal appearance, medications heal open areas and greatly improve itching.

In some cases, LS just seems to come and go on its own. We have learned that surgery is not a way to cure lichen sclerosus, because it tends to come back in the same area. On the other hand, we do know that a shrunken vaginal opening can be surgically widened, and it will heal afterward.

What are some of the treatments?

HIGH-POTENCY TOPICAL STEROIDS

Strong cortisone creams or ointments are a new and effective treatment for lichen sclerosus. They are especially helpful if the skin is thick and/or there is intense itching. Early lesions of LS sometimes heal completely with super-potent topical steroids, while older lesions may just stop itching.
Apply high-potency steroid creams or ointments carefully according to directions and only to the affected areas. The medication can irritate normal skin on the vulva, which can then sting, burn, or become very red. You usually "wean off" the high-potency cream by using it every other day or less, or by using a cream that isn't so strong. Use a strong cortisone on the skin only for control of symptoms. If the skin is not itching, then you should not apply the medication as often.

PATIENT INFORMATION – LICHEN SCLEROSUS *continued*

TESTOSTERONE OINTMENT

For years, the standard medication for LS was testosterone propionate 2% in petrolatum. This is much less popular now because of better results with high-potency cortisone-type creams and ointments. If your doctor prescribes testosterone ointment for LS, apply it to the affected area once or twice daily so that you and your doctor can see whether it is going to help or not. It may take up to two months before the skin becomes less likely to split or tear. If there has been no improvement in two months, stop using the testosterone.

Side effects of testosterone include facial hair growth or deepening of the voice. Clitoral swelling can be uncomfortable if the skin in this area is scarred from LS. If this happens, decrease the application to every other day, then twice weekly as LS comes under control. As the LS improves, apply the ointment less often. It can usually not be stopped completely, however, since LS seems to be a chronic condition.

PROGESTERONE OINTMENT

Progesterone ointment (100 mg per ounce of vehicle) was recommended instead of testosterone for children with LS. There are very few side effects with topical progesterone, but it's no safer or better than hydrocortisone cream for childhood LS.

HYDROCORTISONE CREAM

Plain 1% hydrocortisone cream or ointment is often very helpful for children with LS, especially if they are itchy. (Of course, you should take the child to the doctor for a diagnosis before treating her.) Adults with mild disease may get relief from itching with hydrocortisone, but treatment with higher-potency prescription medications is usually necessary. Hydrocortisone cream or ointment is safe to use for months, unlike the strong prescription creams.

Can LS develop on other parts of my body?

Most patients with lichen sclerosus only have it around the genitalia (and often the anus), but in some cases, it appears on some other areas of the body. Patients who get widespread LS usually have it on other areas of the body from the beginning. Patients who have had only genital lesions for years are less likely to develop LS elsewhere. The typical skin lesions are flat white or pale "confetti" spots that may gradually come together and enlarge. While they can occur almost anywhere, they rarely involve the face.

What would happen if I got pregnant? Could I have a vaginal delivery?

LS behaves differently in different patients during pregnancy: some have fewer symptoms, while others report more itching and discomfort. LS shouldn't prevent a vaginal delivery, and stitches should heal as well as in other areas. For symptomatic relief during pregnancy or while breast feeding, hydrocortisone 1% cream is safer than topical testosterone. More potent steroid creams might be used for short periods of time if symptoms are severe, but these are usually not necessary during pregnancy.

Is there a chance that LS can turn into cancer?

Lichen sclerosus scars the skin, and this increases the risk for a local type of skin cancer. (This happens in less than 10% of cases, however.) The signs of a developing skin cancer are similar to those on other parts of the body: a sore or ulcer that doesn't heal in a few weeks, a lesion that continues to bleed easily, or a bump or raised lesion that is getting progressively larger. If these do not heal despite regular use of your prescribed medication, then let your doctor have a look. It may be that your cream or ointment needs to be changed, but a biopsy might help to tell what's happening. This is usually a minor procedure done in the office with a local anesthetic — a small plug of skin can answer many questions for you and your doctor.

What should I watch for?

You should examine the vulva the same as you would any part of your skin — look for changes in pigment or thickening of the skin. You should have regular (at least yearly) visits to a gynecologist or dermatologist who knows about lichen sclerosus. LS is not necessarily a "premalignant" condition, but your doctor should do a biopsy any time he or she suspects that a change might be abnormal.

PATIENT INFORMATION – LICHEN SIMPLEX CHRONICUS
(like-in sim-plex kron-i-kus)
Latin for "thick skin simply caused by chronic scratching"

Is lichen simplex chronicus the same as "vulvar dystrophy"?

"Vulvar dystrophy" is an old name for several different skin conditions. Now we use a specific diagnosis (like lichen simplex) whenever possible, because we have different treatments for each condition. By the way, there are other vulvar skin conditions with the word "lichen" in their name (lichen sclerosus, lichen planus); these have NO relationship to lichen simplex.

What caused my itching? Do I have an infection?

Many things can trigger itching (like a fungus infection, a skin allergy, or just irritation) but usually the itching stops when the skin gets well. If you've scratched for several weeks, however, the itching can continue on its own. The original trigger for the itch usually resolves completely, so there's no reason to keep treating for an infection if the problem is really itchy skin.

Scratching can make itching worse — this is the "scratch-itch cycle." Rubbing and scratching gradually thicken the skin, making the leathery surface we call lichen simplex chronicus (LSC). The skin nerve endings in LSC signal "itch" more often than in normal skin. Over time, it becomes impossible to tell whether scratching triggers the itch or vice versa. Itching and scratching often worsen with stress. Vigorous scratching gives pleasure and relief, and you may even scratch while you're asleep.

Is something else wrong with me?

LSC seems to develop more easily in patients with atopy (a history of childhood eczema, usually with a family history of asthma, hay fever, or dermatitis). Patches of eczema on other parts of the body may mean you have an atopic background. You can get LSC anywhere on the body that you can reach to scratch, but usually there are only one or two itchy areas.

What else could this be?

LSC on the vulva looks like other thick, scaly, itchy skin disorders. The doctor should be certain that there isn't a fungal infection before prescribing cortisone creams or ointments. If you have applied many different medicines to relieve itching, this can cause contact or irritant dermatitis. You must tell the doctor everything you have used (and are using). A biopsy may help your doctor diagnose LSC.

Can LSC be cured?

The goal in LSC is to stop the itch-scratch cycle, because if you can stop scratching, you'll eventually stop itching. It took a long time to develop LSC, so don't expect it to improve overnight. Therapy for LSC consists of moisturizers and mild cortisone creams and ointments for children and potent fluorinated or medium-strength steroid creams or ointments for adults. Antihistamines or sedatives may relieve nighttime itching. Oozy or moist LSC can become infected, so you may be given oral antibiotics and/or vaginal antifungals to encourage healing. Surgical procedures and alcohol injections are not necessary for LSC.

Apply the steroid cream twice daily for the first month, then daily for the second month to control inflammation. (Strong creams cause skin thinning and redness if continued for too long.) Apply only what the doctor prescribes and follow directions carefully. Rub the medication in well. If the cream has been on the skin for at least half an hour, don't worry about wiping it off with toilet tissue. Bouts of itching gradually become shorter, less severe, and less frequent. Don't be discouraged if improvement takes several weeks or if itching flares up from time to time. As the skin improves, taper the dosage with less frequent applications (2-3 times weekly) or less potent medications as prescribed by your doctor. Usually hydrocortisone 1% is safe for daily maintenance therapy as needed.

From Black, McKay & Braude: Color Atlas and Text of Obstetric and Gynecologic Dermatology, *Mosby–Wolfe, London 1995 © Times Mirror International Publishers Ltd.*

Index

Entries in bold indicate illustrations

Entries in bold indicate illustrations